THE
REALITY
CHECKUP

THE REALITY CHECKUP

FINDING THE PERFECT NON-PERFECT VERSION OF YOURSELF

DR. ANDREW ROCHFORD

NEW
HOLLAND

CONTENTS

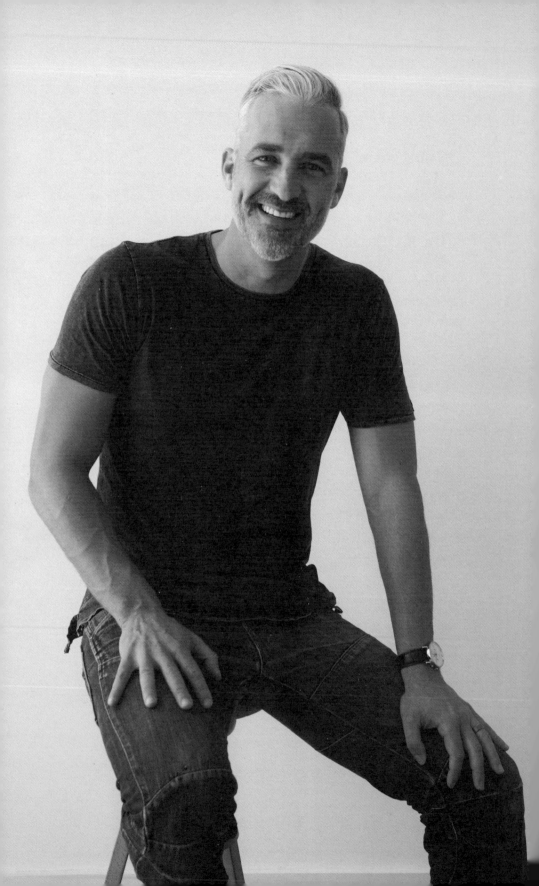

INTRODUCTION

Have no fear of perfection—you'll never reach it.

Salvador Dali

In modern day life, there is a drive for perfection. It's unrelenting. Everywhere you turn there is pressure to achieve perfection. We're not perfect. None of us. No matter how many filters we apply, or diet plans we sell, or stories we tell, perfection in health and wellness is a myth. It took me a while to come to that thoroughly unsurprising realisation, but the good news is perfect 'non-perfection' is both realistic and attainable. And maybe that's what we should all be striving for.

How do you create the best non-perfect version of yourself? Well that's kinda the point of this book. To try and help you answer this question.

I believe that striving for perfection, especially in this very materialistic and outward-looking world, is having a damaging effect on everyone. We are constantly putting ourselves in a position where we feel like we have to be perfect, whether it's at work, in relationships, at home or on the sporting field. We are putting so much pressure on ourselves trying to promote the best version of ourselves when, in reality, there is no perfect version. There is you. And when it comes to health and wellness you are constantly evolving.

For many, including probably me at points, striving for perfection is really striving to cover up our insecurities. And it's that constant pressure that can have a huge impact on your health—your mental health, your physical health, every type of health.

My message is it's okay to admit you aren't perfect.

But how do we become the best non-perfect version of ourselves? How do we overcome the mistakes we all make? What are the things we can do better that we don't necessarily know about?

We all want to make the perfect health choices. That's the first mistake. No matter what blog, or online post you have recently read, there is no 'one size fits all' perfect set of health choices. If you want to have perfect health you'll always fail. There is no such thing as perfect health— there are too many things that are out of your control— and failure to achieve that impossible state is really about people setting unrealistic goals for themselves.

Now this doesn't mean I'm prescribing that everybody gives up, What I'm trying to explain in a round-about fashion is that, there can be a very good, very healthy (yet non-perfect) version of yourself. There are always things you can do better, especially when it comes to your health, who you are, and your wellbeing.

There is no such thing as a perfect game. Taking that sporting analogy a little further, life is the one 'game' we all play. We make decisions every day that impact our performance, especially when it comes to decisions about our health and wellbeing. Now more than ever people will impart (or sell you) advice about how you can 'play' the perfect game but how can that be when we are all so different? Well, that's the point; it's actually not true. There is no perfect game, no perfect way to live life. Mistakes are made, but we can learn from those mistakes.

There are things that I have learned along the way, knowledge that I have gained. I am someone that has been fortunate enough to have seen many things in the world of health and medicine. But I am not the guy who has all the answers—I have taken a long time to realise some things about myself—but in recent years I have come to understand that everybody is trying to sell you something. How to live longer, have better-looking skin or be better in the bedroom.

Life is not quite that simple. Everybody is different. Everybody has their own blueprint—the genetics they inherit from their parents, their lived experience.

TAKING IT A BIT EASIER

I'm in a glass case of emotion.

Ron Burgundy

I want to give people the opportunity to give themselves a break. Life is hard enough as it is without me making you feel worse with yet another book that points out all the things you know you should be doing, but just haven't got around to yet. So read, gain knowledge, reflect, and don't feel bad. Feeling bad in health gets you nowhere.

I believe once you're able to understand that none of us are perfect, and that you have to be able to give yourself a break, you improve your chances of better health rather than hinder them.

Here's an example. You decide enough is enough and it's time to start eating healthy food. We've all been there. That inner monologue that usually kicks in the morning after eating an entire frozen cheesecake or block of dairy milk by yourself. Don't be ashamed, I've done it. And, if it makes you feel any better, research out of Barcelona's Bellvitge Biomedical Research Institute in 2014 cited that sugary sweet food such as chocolate stimulates that the ventral striatum part of the brain triggering positive emotions, similar to those activated by sex or drugs. So, don't beat yourself up.

But anyway, you've once again decided better food choices start from right now, and You have battled through the first few days to almost get through a week and the weekend arrives. Just as you start to feel good about yourself, you inhale an entire ham and pineapple pizza. Now for most of us the moment the last piece of cheesy crust settles in your bloated tummy is the exact point you give up. You feel like a failure. All that week's good choices, wasted. But, that's expecting perfection, and as I've been banging on about, that doesn't exist. You have to realise that you are still seven days further along than you were a week ago—sure you probably could have pulled up a few slices earlier, but eating pizza shouldn't be the end of the world for you.

And that's the whole idea behind this book. Set yourself achievable goals and give yourself realistic feedback.

Until we pause for a moment and admit that the current direction of health, wellness and fitness is leading us towards an unrealistic and, in a lot of cases, an irresponsible version of ourselves, we are actually making things worse.

I want the people who pick up this book to get an insight into how they can live the happiest and healthiest life they can within the bounds of reality, understanding that there are things we know now that we didn't know 100 years ago. That knowledge gives us a much better chance of living a longer life. There is now a better understanding of how we should exercise, what should we eat and how much sleep we need.

Unfortunately, we have created a health, wellness and fitness space for ourselves that is so full of misinformation that it is very difficult to find out anything useful. The problem is not so much finding the right answers. The problem is creating expectations of ourselves that are unrealistic, which leads to perceived failure, feeling bad and a lot of the time giving up.

I don't have all the answers, far from it, and all I can hope is that by the end of this book I can impart some of the things I have learnt so that you can be better equipped to be a better 'non-perfect' version of yourself than you were at the beginning.

THE IMPORTANT STUFF

There are more important things in life than winning or losing a game.

Lionel Messi

For men of any age there are many important issues, but at the top of the list are sleep, exercise, work, relationships, stress, mental health, knowing your body and a few other bits and pieces. This book is about giving you practical steps, based on background research and above everything a commonsense approach, to achieve the healthiest non-perfect version of yourself.

Imagine there was a device that could measure your contribution to your health like the Scales of Justice statue. Every day you make decisions that tip the health scales of your life one way or another. What am I going to eat for breakfast? Am I going to take the bus or walk to the station? Am I going to have a couple of beers after work or head to the gym? We should be trying to make the right decisions without being fixated on extreme diets, unrealistic exercise plans or some magic pill.

It's not news to anyone that we don't move as much as we

once did. There was a time when life was very different. We had manual jobs, getting from A to B took more effort than a couple of taps on a phone app. There was no electric lighting or beautifully designed electronic toys to keep us up at night. The food we ate fell from trees or was pulled from the ground and was prepared fresh and unprocessed. Now, I am the last person to deny the hugely positive advancements mankind has made; I am a self-proclaimed innovation groupie, but I think it's important to note that on the way to the holy land of UberEATS, Netflix and drive-through bottleshops we have created a world that makes being healthy a lot more tricky.

As humans, our physiological and biological evolution in the past century has been modest but mostly in keeping with what the 'father of evolution' Charles Darwin would have expected. However, our social situation, how we co-exist, how we live, has changed at an incredible rate.

The irony today is that in spite of medical advances, research into optimal exercise techniques and our ever-growing knowledge base about all the different foods we eat, our changing work places, and especially the influence of technology, have made our lifestyles more sedentary. Something has to give, and sadly it appears to be our health, physical and mental.

If you posed the question, 'What's the perfect breakfast?' to 10 different nutritional experts, some actual and some self-styled, you may get lucky, and have them come back with one or two points of consensus on a few key things. This much protein, this much whole grain, this much of this one, this much of that one. But you will never get a 100 percent agreement. That has pros and cons. Pro—none of us are the same and there shouldn't be a one-size fits all approach to anything in health. Con—well a lot of the time, a 'con' is exactly what it is.

Many will cite some form of latest 'research' that supports claims of the life-lengthening benefits of a morning elixir of goat's blood and urine. Okay. Fine. There probably isn't anyone claiming that a breakfast of goat's blood and urine makes you live to 150 with the sex drive of 20-year-old. But be honest, there was a moment there you considered whether you would be able to stomach such a 'research' backed panacea.

And that is a big part of the problem; it's really easy to say the words 'research shows', because honestly, who has time to check? Especially with all the busyness of breeding goats and storing urine.

The philosophy of this book is that if you're looking for that kind of 'magic-bullet perfection' you will fail. However, if you go for the best non-perfect, realistic breakfast, you actually set yourself up to live a life that's not only healthy, but maybe even a little more palatable. You'll be as healthy as you possibly can be, and you'll be pursuing a realistic goal.

I hope this book will build self-awareness. You need to understand what your body can't do and, at the same time, know that you can feel better about yourself by doing something else. It's about giving yourself permission to try incremental changes—not seeking to be like everybody else, allowing yourself to seek improvement not perfection.

The idea is to have small wins. I am not the authority

on exactly how people should live their lives. I'm actually trying to help people achieve small victories. Lots of them. As many as we can possibly cram into a book.

I hope that by the time you reach the end of this book, you feel you are in a better position than you were when you started reading. I hope you won't be feeling overwhelmed any more, you will be able to be confident enough in yourself that it's no longer about the attainment of some version of perfection that the world is trying to create, but about the attainment of your own version of perfect non-perfection. I'm hoping you will have shifted the scales just enough.

My hope is that this book empowers people to understand that their health should not be about seeking perfection. But it's not about giving up either. It's about empowering yourself with the knowledge and motivation to strive for healthfulness every day, without feeling the added pressure of unrealistic goals. Being as healthy as you can be is hard enough without the added weight of 'perfection'.

Trying to look like the guy, or girl, on the cover of the health magazine, shouldn't be anyone's goal, because believe me, that guy or girl doesn't even look like that.

Finally, Before I dive into all the good stuff, one last thing. I want you and I to make a deal. A deal that I think will help both of us get the most out of this book.

I can't write a book titled the 'reality checkup' unless I'm willing to bring a few of my own realities to the table. Truths about the mistakes I've made, the things I've ignored and the tough lessons that I've learned. So, the deal is, I'm willing to reflect on my health, mental and physical, as long as you're willing to do the same. It's as simple as that.

Health and wellness requires a level of selfishness. Now I'm fully aware that selfishness is an unpopular, ugly word, but it's the truth. Unless you care about your own health first—by definition be 'selfish'— then you will never be well enough to fully look after others. So, if we can agree on that, and we agree on this book being about discovering the best non-perfect version of yourself, then we must start with the self-truths.

How hard do you push yourself when you exercise... really? How much do you drink...really? Have you ever been depressed...really depressed? Have you ever had a pain in your chest you can't explain? You get the idea.

The truth is, unless you're willing to be honest with yourself about your health you'll only ever achieve part of what you're truly capable of. So, we have a deal?

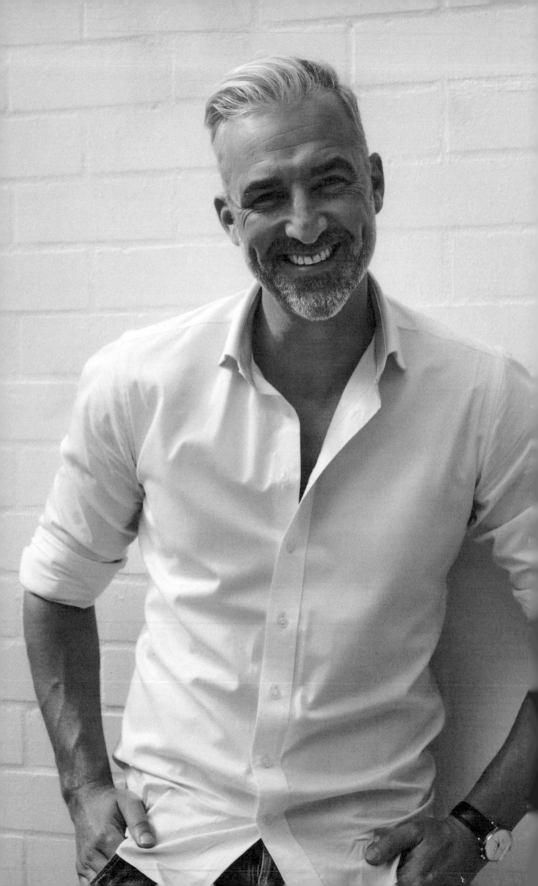

MY STORY

Since I was born, I've done some stuff.

Dr Andrew Rochford

We were and still are a big family. I was the second of five and I was always a competitive kid (that's an understatement). I had talented siblings, all driven to achieve something in life. Education was important and Mum and Dad made sure we did our homework and studied hard. They also made sure we ate well. We had lots of home-cooked meals and in most cases, there was a swag of vegetables involved—stuff I hated, the good stuff, like squash, broccoli, pumpkin and cauliflower. I wouldn't say I was a fussy eater, but I still remember on more than one occasion, in my early years, being left to sit at the dinner table for hours after dinner was cleared. I can still remember forcing myself to last through a full cycle of the dishwasher before I would succumb to having to eat my vegetables. Now, in the years since becoming a father—my kids are now nine and ten—I can't help but chuckle to myself at the memory of staring down a belligerent four-year-old (two, usually, as I was blessed with twins) who refused to eat their beans. Don't worry, I have a full grasp of the 'genetic' irony that their gustatory fortitude was likely my doing, but when you become a parent, your memory becomes very selective and your rationale very sound: 'That soggy, overcooked eggplant may taste like torture, but I make you eat it because I care.'

Sure, I try to carry on the teachings of my mother and father, but parenting 30 years ago was different. I'd like to say it was more militant, but I can already hear the voices of generations past moaning, 'Militant? Please! You had it easy, my parents made me forage for seeds, plant my vegetables, nurture them, protect them from frost, harvest them, clean them, peel them, cook them, and only once I had done all that was I given the privilege of eating them while I walked to school barefoot in a blizzard.' Okay, fine. My parents were firm but not extreme. You ate what was put in front of you and you had to sit at the dinner table until you finished your meal, that was that. We had treats too, maybe a pizza or, most amusingly, soft drink. Picture five children age between two and ten lined up at the kitchen bench watching Mum measuring out the No Frills soft drink—and when I say watching, I mean glaring. Five sets of beady little eyes fixated on the weekly sugar rush. I don't want to use the term 'junkies' but looking back now it did have a little bit of the *Trainspotting* feel about it. 'Choose Life. Choose a job. Choose a career. Choose a family. Choose the biggest f**king glass of No Frills lemonade.' I can imagine it was quite scary for my mother, because had she erred even slightly at that moment, shrieks of injustice would ring out. Such was the drama of Friday night soft drink in the Rochford household.

I've come to realise how lucky I was to grow up on the northern beaches of Sydney. The beach was and still is my happy place. We were at the beach as often as we could. I still love coming home after a day of being dumped by the waves, jumping in a warm shower and discovering all the sand that has found its way into places I didn't even know existed.

Being active was just part of being a kid. Relatively speaking, there wasn't a lot of TV in our house. This was mainly, because we only received two channels, the ABC and NBN from Newcastle. We couldn't get the commercial channels. The upside of my TV-deprived childhood was a lot of time spent outside. I still remember spending an entire summer with my brother constructing what can only be described as the treehouse to top all treehouses. We hammered stairs into the trunk, different branches supported all the different 'rooms', I vaguely remember an attempt to implement a flying-fox escape hatch. Let's just say our imagination and construction prowess weren't entirely proportionate. We would even have slept up there if we weren't a so certain of the existence of werewolves.

Being a kid was fun; exhausting, but very fun. When we weren't up a tree or digging a fort, we played a lot of sport. Endless hours of hitting, throwing, and catching a ball. Didn't matter what shape the ball was as long as there was a competition, and I, as the older brother, went first. We never spent much time sitting around.

I don't remember the exact moment I decided to get into health and medicine, I just remember always being fascinated with how the human body works. Dad was a pharmacist, Mum was a nurse, and their influence only made my path into the medical sciences easier. My dad was diagnosed with type one diabetes when I was about two. High doses of steroid to treat his inflammatory bowel disease had the unfortunate side effect of destroying the insulin producing cells in his pancreas. When you are about 10 years old and you're holding your dad's hand while he is having a hypoglycaemic seizure in the middle of the night and your mum is calling the ambulance, I guess you develop a keen appreciation for the world of medicine.

My dad's illness and the way he dealt with it has been nothing short of inspiring. Life is harder for anyone living with a chronic disease. There is a discipline that is required the rest of us don't have to worry about. Remaining disciplined every day is the difference between staying on top of a chronic disease, and it getting on top of you.

He ran every morning (most days he still does, at 70) and he is only one of the remaining four or five people who have run in every *Sydney Morning Herald* half marathon. He ran his own community pharmacy for nearly 30 years, raised five kids (with a significant amount of input from our amazing mum) and has had plenty of ups and downs. But still to this day I have never once heard him bemoan the health conditions he has had to manage. He has just gotten on with it. Watching this I have gained an incredible understanding of how the decisions we make every day directly impact our health. For him the difference between a little too much insulin, not enough food, too much food, not enough exercise, too much exercise and not enough rest can all have catastrophic outcomes. For most of us, it's a lot less extreme, but still an important reminder of the impact everyday health choices can have, both positive and negative.

It's important to have strong influencers in your life. And as I write this, I am still coming to terms with losing one just recently, my 97-year-old paternal grandfather, who we all knew as 'Grandad'. As a kid, he (and my maternal grandfather, Pa) were both larger than life characters. Grandad lost his left arm from below the elbow in the merchant navy in his twenties; well, at least that's the story I was told. Since my children were born, I have also overheard him telling them other versions of the event. It was lost during a fight with a bear, caught in the door of a school bus, eaten by a monstrous fish during a fishing expedition and run over by a train. As I said, he was a character. Irish born, cheeky, quick-witted but firm. He was a builder, one of Sydney's earliest developers. If you've ever driven around Sydney you have likely passed one of the many blocks of units, schools or houses he was responsible for building.

He also built a couple of boats, including a 30-foot yacht he built in the front yard. I remember as a kid climbing inside the timber framework of the hull that always made me think of the ribcage of a whale. Once inside it was the job of my brother and I to hold nails while he hit them in—

remember, he only had one arm, so he couldn't hold them himself. I would shake like a leaf holding those nails tweezed between the very tips of my fingers. Every time he swung the hammer I would flinch and get my fingers out of the way as fast as I could. And every time he would connect flush with the head of the nail and drive it through the timber with just one blow.

That memory of him then is in sharp contrast to his circumstances over the last five or so years, in a care facility, shuffling from chair to bed, struggling with dementia until he peacefully passed away.

My mother's father, Pa, was also a character. A man of the land, more so than the sea. He always had a coup full of chooks, an aviary full of finches, the odd sheep, maybe a goat and his trusty Staffordshire bull terrier by his side.

I still remember the day he showed me his 'snake whip', a twisted length of steel rope, two-fingers thick, a metre and a half long and curled into a loop at one end to form a handle. To a 12-year-old it looked scary, almost medieval. But as Pa would say, 'It's not as scary as a three-metre-long brown snake latched onto ya ankle.'

We would walk in the long grass beside the golf course near where he lived, socks pulled as high as humanly possible, looking for stray golf balls. As we walked he would casually swing his whip by his side, always at the ready. Now, I never did see him use it. In fact, we never actually saw a snake. And still to this day, I question whether it really was a 'snake whip', or just an old piece of metal cable and a grandfather having a bit of fun with his gullible grandson. Pa died in his seventies of bowel cancer. He, like my grandad, reduced to a skeletal shadow of his former self. Another cruel example of the frailty of life and the blunt contrast between illness and health.

On reflection, it's important to get the most out of your life while you can, because every day that passes is another day you don't live again. But that doesn't mean you can't get the most out of the next one.

By the age of 17 I'd figured out I wanted to be a doctor, which meant getting a leaving mark of 99.9. Ironically, at the same time I was smart enough to understand that 99.9 was a really high mark, I wasn't actually smart enough to get it. But that didn't stop me from giving it a shot. I knuckled down and did my best. But I also didn't give up on the other parts of my life that I loved. Sex, drugs and rock 'n' roll. Alright, I may be embellishing my level of 'cool' slightly. So, let's go with sport, mates and the odd sausage roll.

I didn't get that mark, but I got a pretty good one, and decided it would be post-grad medicine for me via an undergraduate degree in medical science, majoring in anatomy and neuroscience.

Medical school was fun, at the time it was stressful, but reflecting now, I realise how lucky I was to be studying, and not in a full-time job. Not that I have anything against work, but no-one sits you down and REALLY spells out what having actual responsibilities looks like. You know why? Because if someone came up to you in your early twenties at a house party, or seedy dance club and said, 'Hi Andrew, just want to gives you a quick heads up that when you start full-time work the world is going to need you clean shaven, with an ironed shirt and up-to-date tax returns,' you would still be chugging beers, avoiding growing up for as long as you could. But that's not how it works; we all have to grow up at some point.

For me, that came with a rush when I somehow found myself on *The Block*, in my final year of medicine. I was 24— the youngest male on the show by 10 years. Reality TV was the last thing on my mind. I'm a competitive person and I like a challenge. My wife Jamie and I (we weren't married at that stage) stretched the truth just a bit to get on TV. We may have led producers to believe we had more renovating experience than we did, because we actually had none. I'd built a phone table. And it wasn't just any phone table. It had two shelves, a glass top, hand rail balusters for legs, it was lacquered. It was a mighty phone table.

I didn't take too much time thinking about what I was getting into. I came to understand it was a game built around how much the producer could get one person to annoy another. Not to oversimplify reality TV, but the point of it is to entertain, and conflict is entertaining. I had a great time because I think I was too naive to really buy into the drama, and I guess I wouldn't be writing this book if I hadn't ended up there.

TV wasn't what I was going to do. I was going to be a doctor. I have seen the inside of the body. Literally. I've seen most of the pieces, in the living and the dead. That sounds macabre, but that's how you learn about the layers, the connections, the tissues, the vessels all the interconnected pieces that work in harmony to keep us all ticking over. I'm fascinated by the tangible nature of how muscles work and how bones are connected by tendons and ligaments, how the lungs breathe, the heart pumps, the gut digests and the brain thinks.

Initially, I went down the surgical path and became a surgical trainee. I've been lucky enough to be involved in many operations. I've operated on brains, performed amputations, fixated bones, helped replace joints, removed appendixes and gall bladders. Medicine is like the military. You do your training and you gain experience to rise through the ranks.

I moved from surgery to emergency. It was the medical specialty that felt like it suited me most. When the ambulance arrives, the clock is ticking. You have to be a detective, it's up to you to work out what is wrong, all whilst stabilising the patient and organising the right investigations and treatments as quickly as possible. It's probably something I miss doing. I like to think I was pretty good at the trauma stuff. You have to have self-confidence in that scenario and, on reflection, there were times when I thrived on the pressure of a crazy Saturday night as the registrar in charge. There were nights when it all went well, and there were nights when it didn't.

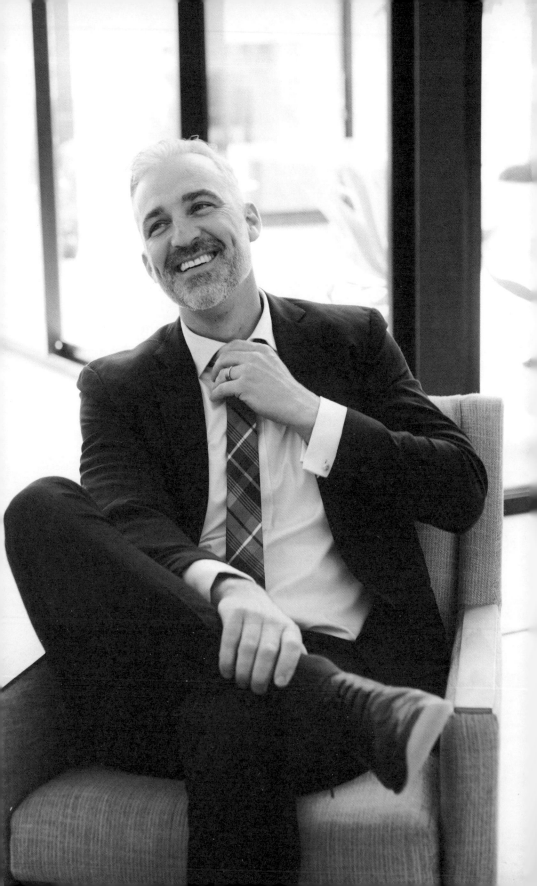

LIFE'S SECRET PLAYBOOK

Everyone has a plan 'til they get punched in the mouth.

Mike Tyson

What makes a champion sports team, or a winning individual athlete? The obvious answer is that they're good at what they do. They're fit, they think fast on their feet and their minds are set on the multifaceted task of winning. But there are two other factors that many spectators, left in awe of their sporting heroes, don't see—the planning and practice that help to make up a prize-winning formula.

The secret in a lot of cases is their playbook—the master plan behind their success.

Let's take basketball as an example. For those who don't understand the game, a group of players bounce and pass the ball to each other as they run towards one end of the court, where the opposing team jumps around trying to stop the ball from dropping into a high basket. It can look like a jumbled mess to the uninitiated but at the elite level every move has been carefully planned by a coach who has drawn up at least 50 combinations of play.

A coach's playbook will contain numerous options that he can explain to his team. Player A can choose to pass to player B or set a screen so player C can get the ball if the opposing team is applying a strong defence. Without a playbook, his team will look like that jumbled mess I've just referred to and their chances of winning the game are inevitably diminished.

Why you ask am I talking about basketball and jumbled messes and plays? Well one reason is to look at this book is as your own 'playbook'—your health playbook, a guide to good management of mind and body. Let this book help you devise a game plan for every day. Help you make better decisions in amongst the busyness of life. The idea is to prep you (like an athlete does before a game) to help you overcome life's greatest opposition (bad health) and prevent an unnecessary early death. That's a dark thought, but it's the truth and that's the 'tough love coach' coming out in me.

It's not about playing the 'perfect game'. It's about maximising health and keeping it at its peak, just like athletes who translate their supreme condition into winning medals. They have figured out all the factors that take them to the highest level. You can be a good dad, a good mum, be successful in business, but all of these things are harder if you have the nagging effects of bad health greeting you the moment you wake up.

I've found that you can talk to some people about maximising their health, but they brush it aside, using any excuse to look into it later. I'm too busy. I need that promotion at work. I'll start thinking about my health later.

The problem is that they might never get that promotion if they're not in shape. Think about how you feel after you've had too many beers the night before. You're hungover, sluggish, tired. You have a funny smell about you. You aren't sharp. You're probably operating well below your potential. The effect is the same if your health isn't up to scratch. You just can't perform to your maximum ability.

This playbook is not intended to steer you towards being a prize-winning athlete; although, if you do achieve that, you will have been paying close attention! Good health is all about playing the health game correctly and efficiently, just as those winning players and athletes stick to a regime before, during and after an event. The 'event' in your case is your life.

The ultimate goal is to get you healthy enough to be at your best in all of your daily tasks. My aim as your good health coach is to leave you feeling victorious over the things threatening to beat you down. If you let things go, if you allow your body to slip, without a health playbook, you'll be exposing yourself to any number of illnesses or, at the very least, avoidable discomforts.

It doesn't matter what your calling in life is, whether you're already fit and healthy—an athlete, even! There will be something in my playbook that will give you a boost and help you to reach peak performance. Whatever your chosen profession, whether you are physically active or chained to a desk, there is always room for improvement. You can optimise your approach for a positive outcome. As your coach, I will endeavour to maximise your abilities, putting you in the best position to perform.

You can't play at your best in life if you aren't healthy.

THE BASICS

Get your facts first, then you can distort them as you please.

Mark Twain

The very basics of good health aren't a mystery to anyone: good sleep, a healthy diet, exercise—the right amount of the right type of each and you're already winning.

There is a commonsense circle. If you get a good night's sleep you have more energy to exercise. When you exercise you make better decisions about the foods you eat. When you eat well you want to exercise more. And when you exercise more you tend to get a better night's sleep. All makes perfect sense, right?

It's a daily lifestyle roundabout and when its working for you everything flows nicely together. When it's not, everything in health feels so much harder.

Patience and motivation are two important parts of maximising your health. Everything in health takes time, which means you need to remain motivated to keep going. If you're out of condition, you can't expect the weight to fall away or your body to reach peak condition after a few short jogs. But it's important to remember that at the end of that first jog, swim or gym session you are in a better position than you were before you started. And the next day, when you find the motivation to head out and do it again, you will again, be a little better off. And so on and so on.

SOURCES OF INFORMATION

We are drowning in information but starved for knowledge.

John Naisbitt

The best thing about the internet is that everyone can be an expert now. The worst thing about the internet is that everyone is now an expert.

The world of online medicine and health is an interesting place, to say the least. But it can also be treacherous. On the one hand, it's the greatest information resource in the history of mankind. You can find answers to all your questions— you just have to know whether you have found the right answer or not. That's the problem, not that the answers are not there. The issue is, do you know whether the answer is the correct one? I keep trying to convince you I'm medically trained and there are times when even I don't know the answer. Can you believe it?!

Medical training is complex and multifaceted. You study (amongst many other subjects) anatomy, physiology and biochemistry, you learn about pharmacology. There is an incredible amount of literature to absorb, examination and diagnostic skills to learn. At the core you learn how to take scientific research information, distil it, digest it and then put it into practice. Doctors are trained to do that. Using the internet as a source of medical advice becomes a problem if you don't understand all the nuances. For instance, who paid for the research? Where did it come from? How old is the research? How large is the study? Are the results statistically significant?

The internet is not a resource to be afraid of—it's a very valuable one. But go into it with your eyes open. You have to understand that while you will get plenty of answers the trick is knowing which is the right one for you.

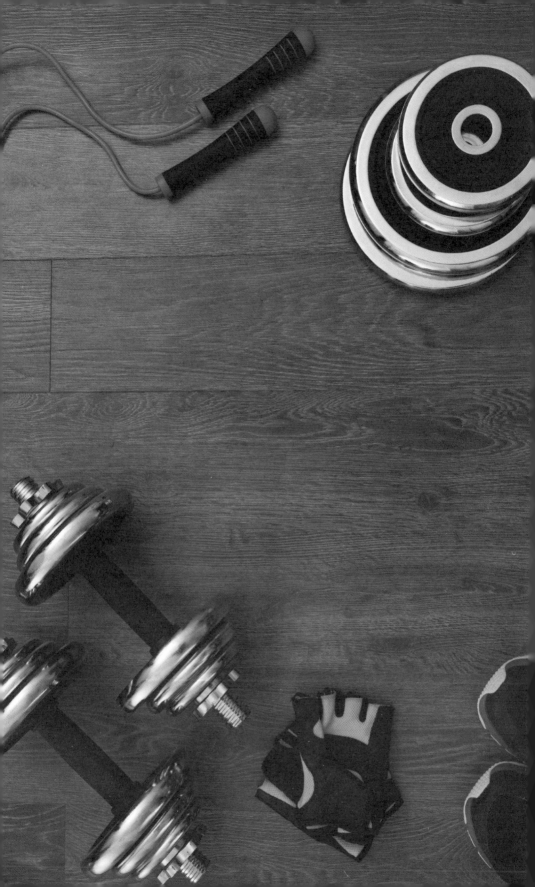

1. EXERCISE

Exercise is done against one's wishes and maintained
only because the alternative is worse.

George A Sheehan

The two vital components for good health management are exercise and diet. Heard it all before? Hippocrates, regarded as the founder of medicine, noted as far back as 400 BC that eating by itself will not keep a man well, 'He must also take exercise.'

So, let me explain why this pairing works.

Physical activity is the very best medicine for mental and physical health. Humans are built to move. From water creatures climbing onto land, learning to crawl, then finally finding our feet and the strength to move against gravity, evolution has gifted us with a biological make-up that thrives on movement. Our hairy ancestors found it more efficient to stand upright in order to move about, using their legs for transport and their arms for finding food, working and building shelters. Every day was full of manual labour, a period of hard physical work necessary for survival.

In our modern world, we still work to survive, but the world in which we exist is very different from the cold caves, sharp spears and hungry sabre-toothed tigers of the past. We work long hours, a lot of the time toiling away at a desk, before sitting in endless traffic to flop down on the couch at night. Or perhaps we don't work hard at all, but still find it very easy at the end of the day to gift ourselves with a 'hard-earned' rest. In the twenty-first century, the number of inactive people is staggering, yet the nature of what we are—living organisms— hasn't changed. We should all be moving more, being as active as possible because that's what we are built to do. I'm not saying we were all necessarily built to move large metal plates around a gym, but none of us were built to sag down into a couch, half sitting, half lying, eating stray Pringles crumbs off our chest in front of a noisy, colourful, flat electronic screen.

To briefly add some scientific weight to my argument, the World Health Organization, in its Global Health Risks study of 2009 stated, 'Physical inactivity (low levels of physical activity) is the fourth leading cause of death due to non-communicable disease (NCDs) worldwide (heart disease, stroke, diabetes and cancers)—contributing to over three million preventable deaths annually (6% of deaths globally).'

'Physical inactivity is estimated to be the main cause for approximately 21–25% of breast and colon cancers, 27% of diabetes and approximately 30% of ischaemic heart disease burden.'

'Physical inactivity is the second greatest contributor, behind tobacco smoking, to the cancer burden in Australia.'

To summarise, movin' is kinda important!

One big problem with our modern world is that technological advancement has seen people standing (or sitting) by while machines and computers do the work for us. And even when we're controlling those computers, it's still necessary to sit down in front of them. The whole point of creating machines to do all the hard, manual work is that we don't have to do it. Who walks to the Post Office to send a letter these days when we can sit at a computer and press a button to magically fire off an email? It's made communication infinitely more efficient, but I can't help but think that the world is a lesser place without the beautiful intimacy of more handwritten letters. And bringing into the argument increasing rates of cardiovascular disease, what could be better for the heart than a brisk walk to the post box to send a romantic, handwritten letter?

Look at the factory floor. Robots are at work, lifting heavy machinery while humans who once pulled chains to lift loads now just press buttons. You could say, technological efficiency is literally killing us. You might think you're being dynamic by saving time and asking the supermarket to deliver your groceries to your door. That certainly saves you time and effort, but what does it mean you are missing out on.

The more you move, the more energy you use, the less likely you are to pile on the kilos, and the more you improve your chances of avoiding chronic disease. Scientists around the world are in agreement that activity literally changes your body and makes it healthier. A good example is an experiment with mice which showed that those which were given a treadmill to run on kept their fur healthy, while those who did not have any means of staying active became lethargic and started losing their fur.

All very interesting, you might say, but humans aren't mice. How can any believable evidence be drawn from the behaviour of jailed mice, forced into an environment where some can play and some can lounge around? Well, it's just another piece of evidence. One day medical scientists will finally succeed in convincing us that activity is the open secret to good health.

An eminent Canadian scientist, who is a strong supporter of the treadmill evidence, is so convinced that good health comes from exercise that every morning he does 200 push-ups before running to his laboratory. Dr Mark Tarnopolsky told *Time* magazine that in studies where blood was drawn immediately after people exercised, researchers found that many positive changes occurred throughout the body. The benefits were an improvement in skin, eye and gonadal health. The gonad, of course, is the sex gland that produces eggs or sperm.

Dr Tarnopolsky recommends 150 minutes of strength and cardiovascular physical activity every week, although very few people manage to achieve that. Not exercising puts you at a higher risk level for different kinds of cancer, heart disease, Alzheimer's, and an early death. The researchers say that when the sedentary mice were subjected to an autopsy they were found to have fat 'all over the place' and half of those tested had tumours. As for the mice that ran on a treadmill, not a single tumour was found. I get it, we're not mice, but most medical research starts with mice, and I think you'd agree, it's not a bad motivator to exercise.

The good news is the growing body of evidence isn't just in mice. More and more research is that there are plenty of compelling reasons to start moving at any age, and even if you're already suffering from chronic illness. Indeed, scientists are learning that exercise is, actually, medicine.

Medical science has advanced, and will continue to advance, creating therapies and medicines for many of the chronic diseases that are so prevalent today. There is no denying that the average life expectancy of humans has been extended by the ability of medication to lower blood pressure, reduce cholesterol, normalise blood glucose and stabilise just about most things. The trap however is using a pill to manage conditions that evidence shows can be improved, or avoided all together, through better lifestyle choices, like regular physical activity. It could be viewed as another form of idleness, adding to an already 'easy-option' lifestyle. Back in the days when medicine wasn't so advanced, doctors would advise those who were sick—leaving aside patients with plague—that physical activity was the best cure. And in today's world, there is a general shift among doctors towards prescribing activity to manage and prevent disease, rather than a bottle of pills.

WHAT ARE THE SPECIFIC BENEFITS OF EXERCISE?

It's simple, if it jiggles, it's fat.

Arnold Schwarzenegger

Let's start at the top, literally, your brain. The more you move the less chance you have of depression, the better your memory and the easier it is for you to learn. Studies also suggest that exercise is, as of now, the best way to prevent or delay the onset of Alzheimer's disease. With current national statistical modelling estimating around 244 people each day are joining the population with dementia, with that number predicted to rise to 650 per day by 2056, now is as good a time as any to start doing everything you can to prevent this horrible disease later in life.

Scientists are yet to pinpoint exactly why exercise changes the structure and function of the brain, but it's an area of very active research. So far, they've found that exercise improves blood flow to the brain, feeding the growth of new blood vessels and even new brain cells, thanks to the protein BDNF (brain-derived neurotrophic factor). BDNF triggers the growth of new neurons and helps repair and protect brain cells from degeneration. It may also help people focus. In a world with so many distractions, who couldn't do with a little help focusing?

I must admit, even before I started studying the science behind exercise and the brain, I always felt mentally more alert and focused during periods where I was regularly exercising.

I always understood that I could use regular exercise to feel physically more prepared every day, and know in retrospect, I was also making myself more mentally prepared.

The most obvious time in my life was getting through med school. I'm not sure I would have made it through without my daily run. Now, you will become acutely aware through my personal reflections in this book that I can be a little obsessive about things. At that time in my life it was running, lots and lots of running. I was never an elite level runner; too big, too heavy, but god it felt good. I think there were probably two main reasons. Firstly, I got addicted to the feeling you get when you physically push yourself to exhaustion. Endorphins flooding the feel-good parts of my brain. And I just loved how it helped me switch off. We all put too much pressure on ourselves at times in our lives. Pressure to get a promotion at work. Pressure to keep everyone happy. Pressure to succeed. At that time in my life it was pressure not to fail my exams. So, the bliss of finding something that was easy for me to do, that helped me, even just for 45 minutes, to switch off from that pressure, became a necessity. Pushing myself to be active, get my heart working harder, red blood cells flowing faster, oxygen reaching my brain quicker, was not only helping me manage my mental health, but it was also helping me think clearer, and pass the exams that were causing the stress in the first place. What a beautiful irony.

And it's not just me...surely, you've felt it yourself at some time in your life. After a gruelling bike ride, a few lengths in the pool or gym class, you get a mental buzz. A lift in the clarity of your thinking, making problems that might normally get you down appear almost incidental and easy to navigate. You feel more relaxed and able to cope with whatever is thrown at you. Countless studies show that many types of exercise, make people feel better and can even relieve symptoms of depression. Exercise triggers the release of chemicals in the brain—serotonin, norepinephrine, endorphins, dopamine—that dull pain, lighten mood and relieve stress. If you haven't felt it, trust me, it's worth giving it a shot. Your brain will thank you.

If the brain benefits of exercise bore you, because you're already working on an intellectual level that us mere mortals could never fully understand, no matter how many spin classes we do, then maybe it's the anti-ageing benefits of exercise that will peak your interest.

Exercise has been shown to lengthen lifespan by as much as five years. A small study out of the Catholic University of Louvain in Brussels found that just moderate-intensity physical activity helps hold back cell ageing. As we inevitably get older—sorry to break it too you but science hasn't figured out how to stop that completely yet—our cells divide over and over again. Telomeres, the protective caps on the end of our chromosomes, get shorter. To see how exercise affects telomeres, researchers took a muscle biopsy and blood samples from 10 healthy people before and after a 45-minute ride on a stationary bicycle. They found that exercise increased levels of a molecule that protects telomeres, ultimately slowing how quickly they shorten over time. Exercise, then, appears to slow ageing at the cellular level. There is still plenty more research needed before Ron Howard is directing an exercise-themed sequel to *Cocoon,* but for now, the findings provide strong support for a way that exercise may keep us young by keeping our DNA young.

It also keeps us looking young. Aerobic exercise revs up blood flow to the skin, delivering oxygen and nutrients that improve skin health and even help wounds heal faster. 'That's why when people have injuries, they should get moving as quickly as possible—not only to make sure the muscle doesn't atrophy, but to make sure there's good blood flow to the skin,' says Anthony Hackney, an exercise physiologist at the University of North Carolina at Chapel Hill. Train long enough, and you'll add more blood vessels and tiny capillaries to the skin, too.

With the modern-day obsession with all thing 'fat', it's probably worth a quick note at this point about one other recent benefit discovered about exercise. It shrinks fat cells. Regular training, of any kind that increases the workload of your heart and lungs, strengthens your cardiovascular system, making it better at delivering oxygen to all the working cells of your body. Burning fat for energy requires a lot of oxygen. A stronger cardiovascular system makes this process more efficient. As a result, your fat cells, which produce the substances responsible for chronic low-grade inflammation, shrink, and so does the inflammation.

HOW MUCH SHOULD I DO?

*If we could give every individual the right amount of
nourishment and exercise, not too little and not too much,
we would have found the safest way to health.*

Hippocrates

This could be the most common question asked in exercise
and fitness: 'How much should I do?' I think that because
deep down we feel like if we ask it often enough, the answer
will get smaller and smaller. In some good news, it appears
modern exercise science has heard our pleading and there
is mounting evidence to suggest that maybe we don't need
as much as we once did. Finally! I hear you sigh, some good
news. But don't be too quick to burn the runners, in health
there is always additional reading.

The Global Recommendations on Physical Activity for
Health, as set out by the World Health Organization is a dry,
60-page document (told you there was additional reading)
but to ensure you spend less time reading and more time
exercising, I have attempted to summarise the important
points for key age groups

For children and young people (5–17 years old)

The bulk of physical activity for this age group must include
play, games, sports, transportation, recreation, physical
education or planned exercise, in the context of family,
school, and community activities. In order to improve
cardiorespiratory and muscular fitness, bone health,
cardiovascular and metabolic health biomarkers and

reduced symptoms of anxiety and depression, the following are recommended:

1. Should accumulate at least 60 minutes of moderate to vigorous-intensity physical activity daily.

2. Physical activity of amounts greater than 60 minutes daily will provide additional health benefits.

3. Most of daily physical activity should be aerobic. Vigorous-intensity activities should be incorporated, including those that strengthen muscle and bone, at least three times per week.

Adults 18–64 years old

Key physical activity for this group tends to be more focused around recreational or leisure-time physical activity, transportation (for example, walking or cycling), occupational (work), household chores, play, games, sports or planned exercise, in the context of daily activities. In order to improve cardiorespiratory and muscular fitness, bone health and reduce the risk of chronic disease and depression the following are recommended:

1. 150 minutes of moderate-intensity aerobic physical activity throughout the week, or do at least 75 minutes of vigorous-intensity aerobic physical activity throughout the week, or an equivalent combination of moderate– and vigorous-intensity activity.

2. Aerobic activity should be performed in bouts of at least 10 minutes duration.

3. For additional health benefits, adults should increase their moderate-intensity aerobic physical activity to

300 minutes per week, or engage in 150 minutes of
vigorous-intensity aerobic physical activity per week,
or an equivalent combination of moderate– and
vigorous-intensity activity.

4. Muscle-strengthening activities should be done
involving major muscle groups on two or more days
a week.

Adults 65 and above

Recommendations are the same as for 18–64 year olds with a
few exceptions:

1. Adults of this age group with poor mobility should
perform physical activity to enhance balance and
prevent falls on three or more days per week.

2. When adults of this age group cannot do the
recommended amounts of physical activity due to
health conditions, they should be as physically active as
their abilities and conditions allow.

What are defined as moderate and vigorous activities?
Moderate aerobic exercise includes activities such as brisk
walking, swimming and mowing the lawn. Vigorous aerobic
exercise includes activities such as running and aerobic
dancing. Strength training can include use of weight machines,
your own body weight, resistance tubing, resistance paddles
in the water, or activities such as rock climbing.

Reducing sitting time is important, too. The more hours
you sit each day, the higher your risk of metabolic problems,
even if you achieve the recommended amount of daily
physical activity.

Short on long chunks of time? Even brief bouts of activity offer benefits. For instance, if you can't fit in one 30-minute walk, try three 10-minute walks instead. What's most important is making regular physical activity part of your lifestyle.

The obvious benefits of activity are firmer muscles, less fat and generally more energy.

But there have to be limits. Overactivity can also lead to problems such as sprains, torn ligaments and general exhaustion. Although exhaustion can hit even the fittest of us if our activities take us beyond the limits of our body's maximum capabilities, the benefits of being physically active outweigh the harms. At the recommended level of 150 minutes per week of moderate-intensity activity, musculoskeletal injury appear to be uncommon. In order to decrease the risks, which are greatest when starting out on any exercise regime, it is best to ease your way into it with a moderate start and gradual progress to higher levels of physical activity

Maintenance of physical activity will keep illness away, especially when we start to wind down as we advance in years. The secret here is not to go into retirement mode, deciding that the days of working for a boss or managing your own company are over and it's time to sit back and enjoy the years that are left. My advice is not to fall into that trap. Even if your work has meant sitting down for years on end, start walking when you leave that office for the last time. It's never too late to start moving!

There are lots of different measures used nowadays to create targets for people to reach on a daily basis. For some it's 10,000 steps, for others 30 minutes. Daily targets can be a successful way for certain people to motivate themselves and fit extra activity into their day. But for others it can initially create unrealistic benchmarks when they are just starting out, in many cases adding undue pressure, leading to failure and giving up. By the way, I would simply advise that to start, look for those moments in the day where you can add more movement—additional incidental activity. This adds up, prepares you for more rigorous targets and avoids you taking the easy way out. Realistically, to reach the levels of physical activity that we were created to achieve on a day-to-day basis, active energy expenditure needs to be both a natural part of your daily life as well as becoming something you consciously set about doing.

Look at it this way, when you sit on the edge of your bed at night before going to sleep, your aim should be to feel like you have done all that you physically could since the time you were in that same spot at the beginning of the day. If you do that day in and day out then your health scales, or at least the exercise ones, will be tilting heavily in your favour.

WHAT KIND OF EXERCISE?

The first time I see a jogger smiling, I'll consider it.

Joan Rivers

You've probably walked past a gym and, through the doorway, seen bulging biceps and heard grunts and groans as dedicated people strive for that perfect body—and the best of health with it. It's a daunting scene for those who have never stepped through that door in the first place, but the good news is that you don't have to start lifting heavy weights or begin to pound the canvas on that running machine. I believe you can maximise your health by setting out to find what works best for you, and what you can honestly see yourself doing with consistency, because consistency is the key.

The key is to find something that motivates you. If going to the gym is an enjoyable experience, carry on. For those who are put off, there are other options. Whatever you choose, focus on consistency and yes, like those who grunt in the gym, try to work up a sweat. No time to do anything because of the demands of the office? Not even taking a break from that computer? Make time. Find a way of introducing physical activity by getting away from that screen for half an hour and walking around the block. On the whole, your physical activity can be incidental or intentional. Whichever, ensure that you indulge in it every day.

Just how much you do depends on your current physical condition and time. If you manage 20 minutes of exercise at the highest level you will derive the same benefits as you would by exercising at a slower pace for an hour. Whatever your exercise goals, the chances of achieving them go up the more you enjoy it and the less mental distress that it brings.

Of course, there are extreme athletes such as big wave surfers, who thrive on mental stress. I wouldn't know, but I'm assuming that's kind of the thrill. And the physical conditioning required to succeed at such a pastime is also extreme. Equally, there are marathon runners—an extremely demanding sport—who push themselves through the pain barrier because of their high-intensity training. They're applying what I would describe as the Whitlam Principle: crash through or crash, a phrase used by the late Prime Minister Gough Whitlam. You can force yourself through the effort, through the pain, and come out feeling physically and mentally fit on the other side. World champion big-wave surfer Nic Lamb put it another way. 'Pushing through is courage. Pulling back is regret,' he said.

Don't push yourself to the point where you are in pain. As Dr Brian Parr, Associate Professor in the Department of Exercise and Sports Science at the University of South Carolina Aiken says, 'The idea that exercise should hurt is simply wrong. Muscle pain during or following exercise usually suggests an injury. However, some muscle soreness is unavoidable, especially if you are new to exercise.'

Here's another idea. Even if you're doing some form of exercise, try to change the intensity—keep your body guessing. Don't allow yourself to get into a comfortable routine. If you walk around the block for three months, same distance, same length of time, your body will switch into easy mode and the benefits will slip away. Take your body by surprise. Keep it guessing by suddenly lengthening that walk or going at a different pace, and even changing up the route so that there is a variety of terrain.

After the devastating earthquake in Nepal in 2016 I flew in with a medical team to help injured people in the foothills of the Himalayas. To give you an idea of the scale of the devastation, in one community every one of the 1700 structures that stood the day before the earthquake had crashed to the ground. It was an incredible journey by road to these remote communities, and what struck me as we passed through each village was that absolutely no-one was overweight.

When I remarked on this to a local medical official he asked me what diseases I had to deal with at home. The obvious answer is lifestyle related health conditions—cardiovascular complaints, strokes and diabetes. For him and the people of Nepal, their biggest issue is communicable disease, infections that we rarely see, or easily treat.

In the West, we have developed medicines to fight these infectious diseases, but sadly, the void of disease is being filled by those related to how we live; sedentary lives with plenty of energy-dense food. In Nepal, people remain active to survive, and the food they consume is unprocessed, a combination creating very different body composition.

It's not hard to feel very fortunate when you see the difference between their lives and ours in the West. And I couldn't help but reflect on how our comparatively 'privileged' life is harming our health. The Nepalese have limited transport, in most cases walk everywhere (an hour from one village to the next and the roads and tracks are all on slopes) carry heavy loads and work the land. There's not a day that goes by when they haven't employed physical effort. Something all of us can probably learn from.

THE REALITY CHECKUP

Q: How much exercise should I do?

AR: You should move—not necessarily exercise but definitely move, move, move—as much as you can, every day. That is the simple answer. The more specific answer is different for everyone. Sure, there are standard guidelines published by the World Health Organization and most government bodies, but the whole idea of this book is that the perfect non-perfect version of you is different from everyone else. Try to cram incidental exercise into every day: walk, squat, jump, carry, dance and lift. Challenge yourself to find the most physical way to fulfil all the day-to-day parts of your life. And do at least 30 minutes of sweat-inducing, intentional exercise as many days as you can each week.

Q: What is the best type of exercise to do?

AR: The answer to that is the type of exercise that you will get excited about doing tomorrow. Consistency is the most valuable element of exercising. If you feel dread at the thought of sliding on the lycra and going back to the spin class then find something else to do. Don't be afraid to experiment. Do it by yourself, do it with friends, do it in a group. Team sport, gym work, swimming and running are good but they are all useless if you don't want to ever do them again.

Q: Should I go to the gym?

AR: Do you like the gym? And I don't mean, do you like telling people you go to the gym? I also don't mean, do you like walking around in a tank top lifting a barbell every five minutes while you catch a glimpse of yourself in the mirror and check Instagram? I mean do you like *going* to the gym? Are you motivated? Do you feel good after you've been? Do you feel like you have worked up a sweat and tipped the health scales in your favour when you go? The gym is a great place for some but not so great for others. The bottom line is you don't have to have an unused gym membership card in your wallet to be fit and healthy.

Q: Can too much exercise be bad for you?
AR: Yes. Especially if you keep exercising on an injury. Health and fitness is a balance, and finding that balance is the key. Undoing it is bad and so is overdoing it.

Q: Is exercise on its own enough to beat a bad diet?
AR: Sadly, no. The two go hand in hand. Many will tell you that to get real results you have to start with your diet. And that is true. Changing your diet in most cases will have a bigger impact on your overall health than changing your exercise plan while continuing to fuel yourself with unhealthy foods. But it does come down to what your goals are. Apply the general rule that no matter what your goal, the best results come from increasing activity and altering your diet in concert with each other. If you filled your car with poor quality fuel it would never be able to perform at its best. Your body is the same; the better the fuel, the better the performance and the better the outcomes.

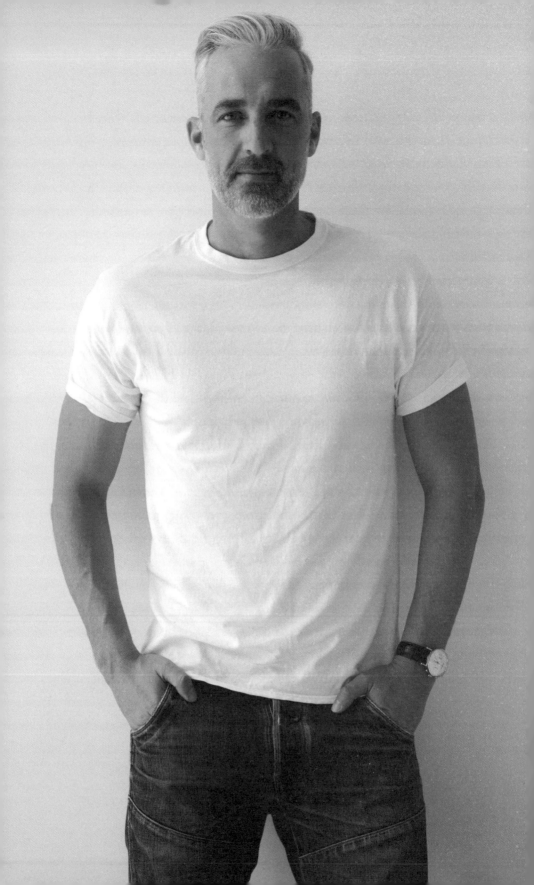

2. BODY IMAGE

People often say beauty is in the eye of the beholder,
and I say that the most liberating thing about beauty is realising
that you are the beholder.

Salma Hayek

So, everyone is happy to agree, society is obsessed with body image. Right? It would seem people are very happy to blame young millennials for this trend. But if you ask me, we are all playing a role.

Young millennials, old millennials, millennial wannabes, those that can't even spell millennial and those who don't even know what a millennial is, share everything. That's a fact. We all love to share.

Just the other day as I was flicking through Insta (that's what the cool kids call it) I stalled my scroll on a pic (again, cool kid lingo) that caught my attention. Staring up at me from my iPhone was a sharply dressed gentleman, wearing a sparkly party hat, holding a sign that said 'I would like 100 likes for my 100th b'day, please'. One hundred likes? Really? I know what you're thinking, just 100 likes? In the world of social adulation achieving 100 likes is a mediocre milestone at best. But that's not all I was thinking.

This man must be one, of only a remaining handful, that were born in the midst of the Great War. This man was 10 when Charles Lindbergh achieved the world's first non-stop transatlantic flight. He was 20 when the Hindenburg exploded; 22 when Hitler invaded Poland; and 28 when 'the bomb' was dropped. This man would have watched Roger Bannister finally break the four-minute mile. He would have been witness to a smiling Yuri Gagarin making it into space. Seen the Berlin Wall go up—and come down. The assassination of two Kennedys, Martin Luther King and John Lennon. The Concorde take flight, the Concorde explode. Man walk on the Moon and man stop going to the Moon. Challenger, Chernobyl and Lockerbie. Mandela in prison. Mandela out of prison. Vietnam and all the Gulf Wars. Tsunamis, earthquakes, hurricanes and floods. This man who was alive, literally, for the birth of the camera, mobile phone and world wide web, was now smiling at me and asking for a quick double-tap between shots of sunsets and perfect soufflés. If he is sharing, it's safe to say it's not just the young millennials.

Instagram Facebook, Twitter so on and so forth, have made it possible to share the world over with just a few clicks. We share everything nowadays, from our breakfast to our opinions and most of all our images. A lot of the time images of ourselves. Now, is that really the problem? Why shouldn't we be able to share?

Alright, let's explore. Is today's modern day body image crisis really the fault of a socially awkward cat from Minnesota posting videos of herself playing keyboard? If you're feeling confused right now, trust me, I will get to yet another one of my unconventional, convoluted points. The answer is probably not. Think how many new friends that cat now has because of the wonders of Facebook. I'm sure it has created a whole new level of self-confidence for Mittens van Beethoven—if that's her real name. The use of social networks has given her a platform to share an otherwise undiscovered gift with the world, thank god. It's all positive for everyone in this scenario. But when does social sharing start to have a negative impact?

I think it starts when the truth becomes hazy. When everyone, including felines, starts posting a version of themselves that isn't real. Sure, a little bit of tweaking with the light, taking a few hundred images before you have the one you want and adding a filter here and there isn't that big of a deal, but imagine I told you right now that Mittens can't actually play the piano, that it's all video trickery and doctoring of images. You'd be aghast, feel betrayed, wouldn't you?

Now, it's okay, calm down, I can assure you that Mittens van Beethoven would never create such a deception, but if she had, an entire generation of moggies would be seriously questioning why they have spent every day fixated on whatever it takes to be just like her.

I am fully aware of the abstract nature of my analogy, but I hope you get my point. If everything you ever see is a version of perfection manufactured by technology, without you knowing, you could easily set yourself unrealistic, unachievable, unhealthy goals, that are impossible to reach. It could easily set everyone up to buy into the idea that you can be perfect.

These expectations are treacherous, because as I said, they make reality hazy. It's no one person's fault, it's just the actuality of the world in which we now live, and being aware is far better than being naive. Nowadays the world wants to see perfect. That's why people spend hours taking photos of themselves, adding filters, editing and enhancing the image to satisfy the expectation of what we feel we should look like. I am the first to admit that I have bought into that. I work in television, the most image-intensive medium, and it's really hard not to start thinking like this.

However, we need to recognise we are setting ourselves up for a pretty big fall. Not only can you be creating an unrealistic set of expectations for yourself, you can quickly fall into the cycle of also not dealing honestly with everybody else. Which fuels the cycle and just transfers the pressure you have felt onto someone else.

It's also important to understand it's not just about competing with editing technology, we all have to be careful not to try and compete with the guys (or girls) you see on the cover of a fitness magazine, a sporting field, in a super-hero movie or body-building website. They work very hard to look like that, it's their job. In most cases they have experienced trainers who understand how to build that physique. Every single muscle has to be tuned so that they look 'perfect', every calorie they ingest is measured, every moment of their day built around how they look—it's the extreme version of fitness and if you ask, many of them will tell you it can be torture.

I figured very early on that I enjoy food. That's an understatement. I love food. Just this past weekend at a family gathering I overheard my mum again telling the story of how my brother and I nearly bankrupted the family with our food consumption during our teenage years. It was not uncommon for us to polish off an entire loaf of bread for afternoon tea. The day we upgraded to an eight-slice toaster I felt like my life was complete. At that time, there was no greater anxiety in my life than coordinating the cooking and buttering of my Vegemite toast with keeping it at the perfect temperature. Oh, how times have changed. Looking back, such an eating regime was ridiculous, and a luxury only a 16-year-old boy playing and training in five different sports teams could get away with.

As time passed, I sadly figured out that I wasn't one of those genetically blessed people that could eat anything and never gain weight. You know the people I'm talking about. Those people in your life that can consume their body weight in deep-fried anything, drizzled with chocolate between two burger buns, never exercise and live with the body fat percentage of a coat hanger. They're not bad people, don't get me wrong, some of my favourite former friends were these people—obviously that's a joke—they were never my real friends. Who knows, maybe you are one of these people, the lucky ones. On behalf of the rest of us I just want to be clear that those looks and comments you get from the rest of us are not about animosity, they are more deep-seated jealously drizzled in spite between two buns of disdain.

The reality of my metabolism became apparent as I transitioned from a teenager who did nothing but play sport to someone who had to start doing other things, like grow up.

There was a time that I carried extra weight—probably 20 kilos more than I should have. It was a slow creep, and looking back on photos, my large frame meant it wasn't ever really that obvious. But the truth is my body composition and weight were unhealthy. From that point on it became apparent that I was going to have to work to maintain the frame I wanted. But it hasn't always been a perfect plan. Body image in the modern world, and the constant pressure for perfection is no longer just about aesthetics, it's become a major health issue—physical and mental.

As a 24-year-old I found out I was going to be on *The Block*. I had zero idea what to expect, but all I knew was that reality TV meant lots of cameras. Looking back now, I know I became obsessed with how I looked. I was fixated on it. Mentally I was in a dangerous place. In the early shots of me on the show I was emaciated. At just over 70 kilograms, with a height of 194 centimetres, I was on the low end of a normal BMI. But I definitely wasn't healthy. I was running, a lot. Every day 10–15 kilometres. Seven most mornings, ten most nights. Those kind of activity levels aren't necessarily unhealthy, but I wasn't eating. I can still remember how hungry I was. I had a constant feeling of emptiness in my stomach. Every morning when I woke up, I felt sick I was so hungry. The irony was, if I had anything to throw up, there were days I felt so sick I would have thrown up. My body was crying out for energy. It went from using stored fat as energy, to using muscle to using whatever it could find. My mind was constantly foggy. Constantly low blood-glucose levels meant I could have slept all day. But of course there was running to be done. It was such an unhealthy cycle I was in. But at the time, I felt as fit and healthy as I'd ever been.

Body image is the most appropriate example of what this book is meant to be about. The misguided pursuit of the perfect body image is fraught with danger. Because what is the perfect body image? Believe me, I was searching for some version of perfect that I wouldn't have even recognised had I reached it. Every time I looked in the mirror, I saw the things I wanted to change. The extra weight that didn't actually exist. Maybe the distortion of what I was seeing was fuelled by fear of being on television, or seeing a body that had carried 20 more kilos than it should in the past. No matter what it was, I can tell you, what I was seeing with my eyes wasn't what was standing in front of the mirror. It was everything else that my head wanted me to see, and that was mostly driven by negatives. You can't always trust what you think you see.

To illustrate my point about how the eyes and mind can deceive, let me explain a physiological fact that you may not be aware of. Much of what you see your brain makes up. That's right, there are parts of your field of vision that get filled in by your brain, not by what you actually see. Allow me to elaborate.

Researchers from the University of Glasgow have shown that when parts of our vision are blocked, the brain steps in to fill in the blanks. The team from the Institute of Neuroscience and Psychology conducted a series of experiments that showed how our brains predict what cannot be seen by drawing on our previous experiences to build up an accurate picture.

The results show that our brains do not rely solely on what is shown to the eyes in order to 'see'. Instead the brain constructs a complex prediction. Dr Lars Muckli, from the University's Institute explains it by saying, 'We are continuously anticipating what we will see, hear or feel next. If parts of an image are obstructed we still have a precise expectation of what the whole object will look like.'

This doesn't entirely explain body dysmorphia, but I've always loved that bit of science and it does illustrate just how much influence your brain has.

Nowadays I'd like to think I have a much healthier body image. Some days I feel good about the way I look and other days I don't. I think if we were all honest it's that way for the most of us. I wish there wasn't any pressure to ever care about the way we look. I'm scared of what the future looks like for my kids given how much it's already changed in my lifetime, but the body image debate isn't going anywhere soon, and that's partly an evolutionary thing.

Let's talk for a moment from the hugely unromantic world of science. The primary reason we are alive is to reproduce and pass our genes onto the next generation, who then reproduce and pass their genes on, and so on (told you it was unromantic). But to give our offspring the best chance of surviving long enough to reproduce, our evolutionary wiring has us choose the healthiest partner we can find—and beauty is often the best proxy for health.

One study conducted in the Netherlands gathered two groups of men and showed them two different sized female mannequins. I agree it does sound a little creepy, but all in the name of science. One mannequin had a waist-to-hip ratio of 0.7, typically considered 'ideal' according to previous studies, and the other had a higher ratio of 0.84, thought to represent the 'average' woman. The two groups of men both showed a preference for the more slender body type. Normally, such a conclusion could be written off as cultural bias, a lifetime exposed to billboards, magazines and every social platform you can scroll through, adorned with images of women that have had the 'waist-to-hip' filter thoroughly applied and present supposedly the ideal picture of body image. But, the clever little wrinkle in this study, that I'm sure had the lab-coat clad boffins of the Netherlands patting each on the back, was that second group of men in the study had been blind since birth.

Do such studies truly answer the debate? I'm not sure. But I do believe the more ways you attack a debate, like body image, the better armed you are to create your own, informed opinion.

It's a bit weird for me to look back and reflect on those periods in my life when I had my own body-image issues. I never really have, and I definitely haven't admitted it was driven by insecurity about my body image. Mainly because when you do everyone has an opinion. And given that body image issues are hugely complex and in a lot of cases fuelled by a fear of the opinions of others, getting more feedback can be petrifying, even if it's positive.

Sadly, I know I'm not alone. On some level, most of us have anxiety issues about how we look on any given day. Some of us are strong enough to cope, others not so much. I'd love to think that there's a way for all of us to help each other, even just a little, starting with the world admitting there is no perfect body. Health and physical wellness needs to be about finding the best non-perfect version of yourself on the outside, and the inside.

I agree, that got a bit deep. But circling back to my original thought about the world of image and breeding and evolutionary science, it's important to remember that our physical appearance and health have always been linked. Since our early days swinging in trees and chasing woolly mammoths, the healthier we were, the stronger we looked, the more lustrous our back hair, the more heads we turned and the better we felt about ourselves. This is of course an extrapolation of what I'm assuming it was like—you can understand there's not a lot of cave drawings that completely outline the body image debate. Biologically speaking we haven't changed that much. We can all still benefit from one of the great side-effects of an active healthy lifestyle. When the inside is healthier the outside bit looks healthier—'better'—as well. And hell, you never know, if you're lucky, you might just get picked up by a blind Dutch guy.

BODY BUILDING

When you're young you think you're bulletproof. It's actually part of the development of the adolescent brain. It takes time for the part that truly understands consequences to be fully developed. Until that happens young men are more likely to take risks: driving fast in a car, trying recreational drugs, or experimenting with things like performance-enhancing steroids There are risks associated with using artificial substances to try and improve anything, or change your body.

If you try and change your body you open yourself up to all the health issues that might be associated with that change. You're manipulating your body in a way that's not necessarily natural. I think it comes back to the conversations around male body image and particularly body image amongst younger males. There is great pressure put on young men nowadays to look a certain way.

What is the perfect body? It's very different from what it was deemed to be five years ago and five years ago before that. Now it's becoming unattainable—it's unattainable perfection. If you start putting those kinds of pressures on men they will try to find a way to respond in the simplest possible way.

When do we decide that we've reached the point where body fat percentage is too low, where muscle mass is too high. Where does that end?

You have to understand why you're doing it. Are you driven by a desire to look like everybody else you see on social posts and on magazines? Is there some other reason you feel your body image isn't perfect, or isn't what it should be?

Your body shape is your body shape. How you look doesn't define who you are. It's not always a reflection of whether you're healthy or not. A lot of textbooks would say that many of these people with 'perfect' physiques actually have very little cardiovascular fitness and are a lot less healthy than a lot of people would expect.

I think that going to the gym or getting outside to be fit and healthy is a good thing but when everything that you're doing is driven by the desire to look a certain way it's not sustainable. What are you willing to do to achieve some level of perfection that you don't even understand? Will you be happy when your muscles are this big? Will you be happy when they're that big?

If you decide to take a shortcut and use some unnatural performance enhancement, then you have to know there are risks.

If you've decided that you're going to use any performance-enhancing drug you'd better understand that you're putting something into your body that can have a negative impact. If you have a professional career, you've got to understand the risk of what you're doing.

Taking certain supplements is not without risk. You should look at what the benefits are. What am I trying to achieve here? What do I want to look like? Where's my end point? Am I doing the right training? Maybe, instead of taking all of these drugs, maybe if I train a different way or eat a different way, or live a different way, I won't have to put my health at risk.

Every decision you make tips the scales one way or the other way when it comes to health. If these supplements are going to improve your health the scales are in a good spot. But do these benefits outweigh any associated risks, including the increased risk of any other disease? Or do I just not know?

There's a multibillion-dollar industry trying to get you to take these supplements. They claim that their supplements are the perfect way to build muscle and to get shredded. The owners don't go to bed at night feeling better because you've got the abs you wanted. They go to bed at night feeling better because they have more money in the bank. Their job is to sell a product. Your job is to inform yourself by talking to people who know.

There are people, nutritionists, dieticians, exercise physiologists and trainers, who take a genuine interest in understanding what you need to put into your body to get a result. Get the right support, the right guidance. Find people that you aspire to be like, who train the way you want to train and have the right philosophy. Talk to them and inform yourself. Align yourself with them—you'll achieve your goals and it's a much safer environment than experimenting on the basis of what you're told by manufacturers.

KNOW YOUR BODY

Take care of your body. It's the only place you have to live.

Jim Rohn

Your body changes as you age. Sorry, it's a fact, one I am really struggling to come to terms with. Many of us who are competitive and have played sport tend to ignore the fact that we are slowing down and don't recover as quickly as we used to. I still play Division 1 basketball with my mates. Guys I have played basketball with my entire life, at all levels. Monday nights is when the competitive me comes out. He's not pretty. In fact, on many occasions he is thoroughly embarrassing. If he wasn't me, there are times I would have questioned his sanity. Seriously, it's only a game.

It's a competitive outlet for me, something that I know helps me physically and mentally, and I want to continue as long as I can. I am scared of the day I can't continue to compete at a level that challenges me. It's part of who I am. Always has been. But that means that I need to look after myself. It might seem silly to some, it's still only social sport, but I know that having that competitive outlet and the drive to not look like a fool out there while the youngsters show me up, gives me a purpose. It's not going to last forever, but I can make it last longer.

It took me a while with different types of training over the years to figure out what works for me. It's important to understand that there are so many ways to exercise and train, and that not all of them are going to work for you. Finding what does is very important. You have to be willing to explore, try different things, work out what works for you.

Something else to consider is injury. Often your life is so full of other things that you don't have time to focus on that rolled ankle, sore back or muscle twinge. You try to forget about it in the hope that it will get better. Or you're just impatient and feel like any hard work you've put in is slipping away with every day you're not training. When you ignore it, or rush your recovery, there is every chance you will actually makes things worse.

My left ankle was chronically painful for five years of my life. There was actually a time when I had resigned myself to feeling the pain for the rest of my life. It started with a couple of sprained ankles that I kept playing on. The type of injury that you can run off during a game, then it really kicks in when you cool down. I'd do almost all the right things. You know how it goes RICE. Rest. Ice. Compression. Elevation. I used plenty of ice, strapping and pillows. My ankle was iced, compressed and elevated up the wazoo (that's a medical term). Trouble is I never did the whole 'rest' thing. Continuing to be active on an acutely inflamed ankle turned it into a chronically inflamed ankle. If you take your fingers and run them over the knobby bit (your fibula) that bulges on the outside of your ankle just before it turns into your foot, and feel the soft gutter just underneath it, that's the exact spot I had constant pain for five years. I was a fit guy in his early twenties who woke up every morning with an excruciating ache right there. When I walked it would radiate down my foot into my little toe. Medically speaking it 'really sucked'. But it's all because I didn't listen to my body. All because I knew better. All because I was a bit of a butthead.

I'd created a 'health economy' that was false. I thought I had to keep going, keep training, keep playing, fight through the pain to stay at my peak level of performance. I felt that if I took a week, maybe two, off to really let the initial injuries heal I would be going backwards. Truth is, a two-week break to let an acute injury heal would have been a far better outcome than five years of underperforming with a chronic injury that wouldn't.

Health is a long game. As I said earlier, you have to be willing to give yourself a break if you miss a couple of days of healthy eating. You also have to be willing to manage how you exercise. You'll need days off to rest. You'll miss days because of other commitments in life. You'll need to recover if you are sore. It's about knowing when the right time is to get back into it.

It is also important to understand that your thinking has to evolve as you age. Many of us hang on to our glory days, just like me. I can't encourage you enough to be active as long as possible. But inevitably, your physiology will change.

Think about that for a moment. What are you capable of doing? What should you be doing? What is the right type of exercise for you? How can you work more activity into your daily routine? When you're older your commitments change. Life can no longer revolve just around your fitness (unless you're a fitness trainer, obviously). You may have family and kids, work commitments and all the other bits and pieces that come with life. Everyone's life is different. Everything has to work together. But that's no excuse.

TAKE CARE OF YOU

*Help me. Help me Rod. Help me, help you. Help me, help you.
Help me, to help you*

Jerry Maguire

One day I was running at Manly, pushing myself up the steps that go over Freshwater. Suddenly I was in pain and having a hard time breathing. I couldn't get up the stairs. For those not medically trained, those are bad signs. Very bad signs.

I'd been getting a few twinges. Every time in the same spot, the left side of my chest radiating into my left shoulder and down my arm. Textbook 'do-not-ignore' kind of chest pain. I had ignored it.

Just for the record, this is one of those moments in the book where I'd really encourage you to apply the, 'do as I say' not 'do as I did' rule.

I'm a trained medical practitioner yet I ignored the pain and put off doing anything about it. I had convinced myself it was nothing. I was only 32, I didn't smoke and I was eating well. There was no strong history of heart disease in my family. It was easy for me to think I was bulletproof. Stupid me.

After the more severe event on the stairs, my inner voice—clearly smarter than my outer voice—finally convinced me to see another doctor, someone who didn't have the incredible bias of knowing the 'patient' so intimately. I went to the doctor, convinced my heart was fine and a few tests would prove that, as always, I was right.

I was in my early thirties, working late nights in Emergency.

Doing TV, radio, speaking opportunities, whatever I was offered. My career was my priority, taking every opportunity, not wanting to say no, or let anyone down. I loved all of it and I didn't have time for anything else. I know I sound like a proper 'hero', ironically, reality would prove I was more of a dill than a hero. By prioritising doing as much as I could for everyone else, I was ignoring looking after myself. I can even remember during an episode of pain thinking, *I don't have time to go to the doctors.* I was really clever.

I wasn't easy to convince, even when I finally started having some tests. The first abnormal ECG didn't do it. A highly abnormal Exercise Stress Test—that's where they wire you up, stick you on a treadmill and make you run as fast as you can, or until you get chest pain—didn't do it either.

The exact moment I figured out I wasn't as smart as I thought I was, I was transferring from a hospital ward bed onto a narrow angiogram bed with my paper underpants-clad arse hanging out of the gap in the hospital gown. It was the most fitting moment. It wasn't a very nice feeling. A combination of embarrassment, fear and anxiety. In hindsight, I was lucky to have reached that point at all. Many people don't get that chance.

Waiting to see the cardiologist for the results of the coronary angiogram took forever. Thankfully the small arteries that supply the muscle of my heart—my coronary arteries—were clear. His explanation, and my diagnosis, was 'effort-induced coronary vasospasm'. A lot of words to say that the blood flow to my heart muscle was being compromised during exercise because my heart arteries were going into spasm. I started medication for a period of time and haven't had issues since.

I clearly wasn't bulletproof, or perfect, no matter how fit I thought I was. I was putting myself in a very risky situation. The pain I was feeling was my heart muscle not getting enough blood or oxygen. That was stupid. Really stupid. The heart kinda needs that stuff. The condition isn't something that was caused by my lifestyle. I have never smoked, always tried to eat good food, and remained active all my life. But none of that mattered. I couldn't have predicted it. Even as it was happening, I didn't believe it had anything to do with my heart. I guess the lesson is, don't ignore the signs, or your own health. You have to put yourself first. You're no good to anyone if your health suffers.

I've always thought that the aircraft safety announcement best captures the idea of looking after yourself. You know that moment just before you take off when the smiling, friendly staff remind you of all the really bad shit that can happen while you're trapped inside a plane—we get it! If anything goes wrong it's fine because you've made us some nice laminated cards to read while we contemplate the size of the crater we are about to form in planet earth; but I digress, again.

During that same announcement, they say: 'In the event of a decompression, an oxygen mask will automatically appear in front of you. To start the flow of oxygen, pull the mask towards you. Place it firmly over your nose and mouth, secure the elastic band behind your head, and breathe normally. If you are travelling with someone who requires assistance, secure your mask first, and then assist the other person.'

'Secure your mask first.' It's sound advice. Look after yourself before you look after others. It's not selfish. It's necessary. On a plane, as well as in life. Something we should all try to follow.

And just briefly, if I'm on a plane and an oxygen mask falls in front of me there is absolutely zero chance I'm going to 'breathe normally', no matter how nice your laminated cards are.

BE PROACTIVE

Action expresses priorities.

Mahatma Gandhi

In health, hoping it will go away is wishful thinking. Dangerous, wishful thinking. Not getting a diagnosis doesn't mean it doesn't exist. A heart attack is a heart attack, even if there isn't a doctor around to tell you you are having a heart attack. Bowel cancer is bowel cancer. A stroke is a stroke. And a mole that is melanoma, is melanoma before you get it checked, just as it is melanoma after you get it checked. You catching my drift?

Putting off seeing the doctor is coming, hugely common. I've just told you about the time that I did it. As you'll recall, just because I ignored something I shouldn't have, didn't make it go away. If anything, I put myself at much greater risk of a catastrophic outcome.

Don't ignore your gut. Metaphorically and literally. Intuition is very important. You know your body better than anyone, so when something is concerning you—really concerning you—there could be a reason good reason why. Also, with an estimated 16,682 new cases of colorectal cancer being diagnosed in Australia every year, noticing literal changes in your guts is also very important.

As a Junior Registrar, I was working a day shift in Royal North Shore Emergency. It was a day like most. Waiting room full of minor scrapes and sniffles. A ward, 50 per cent filled with overflow from the night before and ambulances already rolling in with the day's first customers. On this day, I got to experience an extreme example of what some humans are capable of ignoring when it comes to their health.

Like any other day, I half listened to the semi-coherent hand over of exhausted night staff and hoped something exciting would happen early to fill my day. It didn't. So I started working through the Cat four and fives in the waiting area. 'Cat' means Category. Four and five means, not life threatening at all. Your concern has in fact been deemed so far from life-threatening that we predict you could potentially die from old age before your current complaint kills you, so we are going to make you wait about that long. I'm joking, obviously. Or am I...

Anyway, in most cases it's a sprain, or a cold, or a hypochondriac convinced they have the plague. Standard stuff. Sometimes however if the story from the patient is vague enough, and they appear well enough, something out of the ordinary can get past the incredible triage nurses. On this day a man, or more accurately, his enormous testicle, did.

He was in his late twenties. A well-dressed guy, average height, average build. Average. But his problem was not. He had told the nurses he had pulled a muscle in his groin whilst running, and needed a doctor to fix it. He refused to be examined and all his vitals were normal. He got stamped Cat four. Even that could have been a stretch.

When I called his name and brought him into the examination room it was pretty clear he wasn't telling the full story. Nothing really added up. When he finally got to showing me the issue, it's safe to say I was a little surprised. His right testicle was five times the size of the left. It was like he had a clenched fist inside his scrotum. Not the clenched fist of a small-handed man either. It would have been the clenched fist of a very large-handed man, who had a large-handed father and large-handed mother. Who could never find gloves that fit, and had been a manual labourer his entire life, and had dabbled in amateur boxing. I guess what I'm saying is that the testicle was really big.

When asked how long it had been like that he said 'Eight months.' That's right, for eight months he had been carrying around a testicle the size of a mango. One of the big mangoes. He hadn't seen a doctor. Hadn't told anyone. Just thought it would go away. When I asked him what he thought it might be, his answer was, 'cancer'. At this point I had to explain cancer doesn't tend to just go away. Luckily for him it wasn't cancer. It was a hydrocele. A collection of fluid around the testicle that in his case was fixed with surgical drainage.

There are lots of reasons why men excuse keeping quiet about their health. They don't like to be seen as whingers.

There is that macho thing: it can't be me, that couldn't happen to me. Embarrassment and fear of some stigma which might be associated with being physically unwell. Laziness. Ignorance and even just flat-out indifference: I just don't care. And when you start talking about mental health issues, all of this is much worse.

You can't allow being told you've got a problem to make you feel that you've been marked down on the scorecard of life. If you're striving for perfection that kind of news can be a difficult experience. We need to let go of this idea that we can be perfect. Letting that go is a step in the right direction, to seeking help and improving our chances of solving the problem.

When it comes to those scales of life, making decisions like these are as important as deciding what you eat for breakfast. Your decision will tip the scales one of two ways. Ignore that mole and you are tipping the scales towards a bad outcome. Get that mole seen to instead. If it is a melanoma it gets cut out before it goes too deep—you've tipped the scales the other way; you may even have just saved your own life.

THE REALITY CHECKUP

Q: Should I be concerned about my body image?

AR: No, is the easy answer. But that's a naive way to look at the world and health. You should be aware, but not concerned. How you look is a reflection of your health, and that should be what motivates you to be concerned about your body image, not what other people think. Be proud of your body, be confident and don't let an unrealistic portrayal of 'the perfect body' make you feel less of yourself. But don't use the misguided, mainstream media debate about body image as an excuse for not achieving a healthy, non-perfect physical version of yourself.

Q: Is it narcissistic to focus on my body image?

AR: A large 2009 study estimated that six per cent of people in the United States suffer from full-blown narcissistic personality disorder. But it's likely that many more fall short of the strict diagnostic criteria. By definition, narcissism is the pursuit of gratification from admiration of one's own attributes. The term originated from Greek mythology, where the young Narcissus fell in love with his own image reflected in a pool of water. Do you spend an abnormal amount of time staring lovingly at your own image in the mirror, or reflection in a stream or pool? If the answer is yes, maybe it's teetering on narcissism but it really does come down to your motivations. Why are you focused on your body image? Is it about being healthy or posting pictures and getting 'likes'? Who are you wanting recognition from, yourself or others? Is it creating stress and anxiety and other health problems? Start by being honest with yourself about how important the 'perfect' image of yourself is to you, and how much of your energy you are putting into it. Being proud of the way you look shouldn't be discouraged, but you must understand your reasons.

Q: Should I consider cosmetic surgery?

AR: You should consider whatever you want, but again, be honest about why you are considering it. Are you making the choice for you or someone else? There are so many different forms of cosmetic surgery nowadays, and so many different reasons why people choose to have it done. Judging someone for choosing cosmetic surgery says more about the person doing the judging than the person being judged. Understand your reasons, be sure of what you are hoping to achieve, ask questions, lots of questions, have support, and take your time. Having any form of surgery is significant and there are risks and benefits. The benefits should always outweigh the risks.

Q: How can I achieve beauty perfection?

AR: What is beauty perfection? Can you draw a picture of it for me or give me an example? I bet your example of perfect beauty is different from mine, and mine is different from everybody else's. And I hope it's not all just about the physical. So, the question is, how do you know when you have achieved perfection? I look at it like this, beauty is subjective, hence the saying 'beauty is in the eye of the beholder'. So, when you are the ultimate example of beauty for a 'beholder', any beholder, then technically for that person you have achieved 'beauty perfection'. The healthiest way to unpack that slightly mind-bending analogy is to focus on yourself as the beholder.

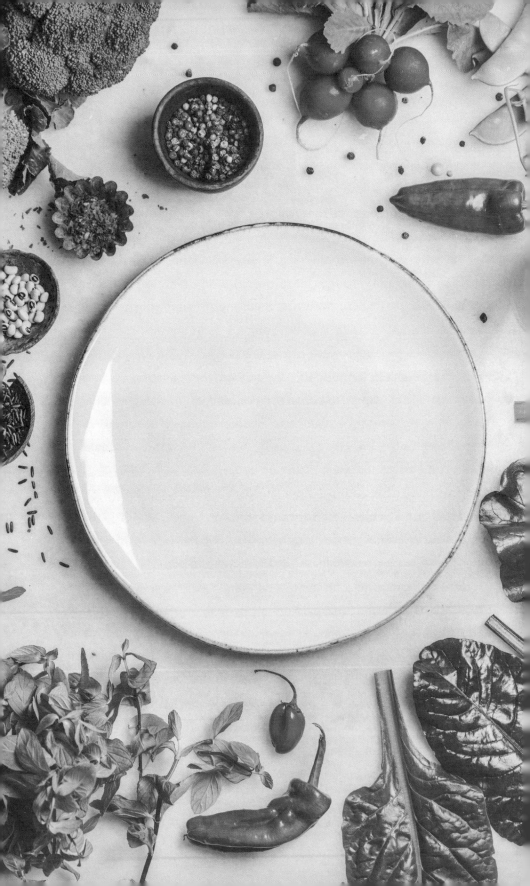

3. DIET

I don't stop eating when I'm full. The meal isn't over when I'm full.
It's over when I hate myself.

Louis CK

———————

Can I start by saying I hate the word diet? Yes, I know it's the title of a chapter in a book that I am writing, but I still hate it. I believe its meaning has become confused. If I was an English professor, or one of those people that play a lot of scrabble, I could give you a thoroughly intelligent-sounding reason why it's confusing, to do with nouns and verbs and stuff. But I'm not one of those people, so I'll just go with my own personal reason for disliking it.

Diet by definition is the food someone eats. Doesn't matter what those foods are, if they are part of the regular foods you eat then that is your diet. The diet of a monkey is bananas; well, they probably eat lots of other stuff but I'm not an English professor and I'm not a vet. For humans, the word diet has been hijacked to always imply a specific fancy regime designed to lose weight. The phrase 'I'm on a diet' invariably means you're eating a specific selection of foods, for a defined period of time with the major focus to lose weight. But we are ALL on a diet. Unless of course you are breatharian—you know, those people that survive just on air. Then again, you could technically argue their diet is air. Anyway, my point is, being on a 'diet' shouldn't just be about weight loss. It should be about the foods you eat, the personal menu you create that has the selection of all the different foods you choose to eat, and the ones you don't. It needs to be about getting into a habit of eating more food that is good for you than bad. If you do have a specific goal in mind, like losing a few kilos, then it's not about 'going on a diet', seeking a whole new alternative to what you normally eat, it's about altering the one you already have. Eating more of this, and less of that. Not eating that anymore and adding some of this. When you start throwing the baby out with the bath water—I obviously don't mean literally, but being hungry can make you absent-minded—and completely switching from one 'diet' to another, you are setting yourself up to fail. Choosing the right foods, losing weight, dealing with being hungry, calculating calories, finding fresh kale, cleaning the juicer etcetera, etcetera, is all hard enough without making your food choices extreme. Am I making any sense? Maybe my blood sugar is a bit low, I think I need some banana bread?

SOME OF IT IS IN YOUR GENES

Let's consider the conundrum of genetics. My grandfather recently passed away at 97. The last of his generation, with all his brothers living into their late nineties and his sister hitting the century. On average, they all lived 15 to 20 years longer than average. It's hard to argue that genetics wasn't on their side. My grandfather wasn't a runner, he ate bacon, lots of bacon, he lived through both wars and most likely he got to 97 because he had 'good' genetics. At the other end of the spectrum, I have had to talk to parents whose kids have died in their sleep because of a genetic condition. There are the extremely fit with sky high cholesterol. Melanomas in places never even exposed to the sun. Smokers that live into their hundreds and non-smokers with lung cancer. There are things in life you just can't influence, like your genetics.

Genetics makes you who you are. It's the bits from you mum and the bits from your dad. It's a lottery, you'll get some good, and some bad. At the time when that is decided you don't get a lot of say, so there's not much point getting upset about it now. The reason I bring it up is because, despite the obvious fact that you can't change your genetics, or how they will impact your health, what you can change is the other stuff. The lifestyle choices. Those decisions you make every day that tip the scales one way or the other. Your life, and especially your health is not a path that is set in stone the moment you begin to exist. You have the chance to make choices that send your health in one direction or another, good and bad.

In my younger years, I paid my way through med school working as an assistant nurse at RSL War Veterans Nursing Home. My mum has worked in aged care, and I have the upmost respect for the profession. So, what better way to get acclimatised to care and medicine that working in nursing. It was a hugely rewarding job, hearing some great stories from men and women that had served our country in many different wars, including one of the last living Anzacs before he passed away. Looking back now, as 19-year-old I'm not sure I grasped the gravity of that privilege. I do now.

Needless to say, my days as an AIN (Assistant in Nursing) weren't all filled with cups of tea listening to stories from Australian heroes. There were some genuinely disturbing moments. I'll never forget the day I was showering Ted. I will never forget poor old Ted. His name is burned into my memory. So anyway, I was showering Ted. He was a kind, wiry, tall man and sadly, as is the case for so many, in the early stages of dementia. To get him from his tub chair into the shower chair required a lifter. It was quite the operation because despite his frame, and lack of balance, Ted was still strong enough to push down on the harness that looped under his armpits, and try to lift himself up and out. Timing was everything. But once he was in the shower chair, Ted was usually very happy. He did enjoy his daily shower.

We had successfully navigated the transfer and I had turned for a minute to wheel the hoist out of the shower when I heard the first scream. It was completely out of character for Ted to scream; as I said, he always enjoyed his shower. The next scream was worse than the first. I rushed back into the shower and the look on Ted's face was pure agony. Absolute pure agony. There he was, sitting in his chair, almost whimpering, with a pleading look of torment in his eyes. But I couldn't see what was wrong. I was expecting to see him on the floor in a pool of blood, or with a deformed limb. But he was still sitting in the chair. No blood. No broken limb. I couldn't for the life of me figure out what it was. I started the shower up, while continuing to look for any clues to what was wrong, because by this stage Ted was beside himself. And then I saw it. I had gotten down on my haunches to take a quick look under the chair, and that's where it was. And the reason Ted now had tears rolling down his face became very apparent.

As Ted was sitting waiting for the shower, he had decided to use his arms to push himself up and adjust his position in the plastic shower chair. It would be a decision he would come to regret. What Ted didn't know was that the flat plastic of the chair, underneath his undercarriage region had a crack in it. So as Ted had dropped his bottom into the chair, the plastic had given way, and forced Ted's entire scrotum—including its contents—through the seat, where it was now trapped. Looking from below, it very accurately resembled the scene from *Something About Mary*, when Ben Stiller's character hastily pulled up his fly and got his 'beans and frank' trapped in the zipper of his jeans. In Ted's case, it was just the beans, and the jagged teeth of the cracked plastic deck chair, were his zipper. You can now understand why I have never forgotten Ted's name. Poor old Ted.

I didn't bring up my time as a nurse to discuss nearly castrating Ted. I brought it up because that was the first time I noticed the phenomenon I call the 'Two Spikes of Life'.

In simple terms, over my time as an AIN and then into the years as a doctor, it's become abundantly clear there is a spike of mortality among people in their seventies and another spike in the nineties. I should probably call them the 'Two Spikes of Death' but that just seems a bit brutal. Basically, it's my very unscientific observation that lifestyles tend to catch up with people in their seventies, and for the genetically more robust they get to their nineties, and survive things you never thought they would. If you're going to die of a heart attack or a stroke then there is a high chance you'll be in your late seventies. But those that get through that, and into their nineties, you can't kill them with a stick! That's obviously another figure of speech, I have never attempted to test whether you can kill someone in their nineties with a stick. I am happy to go on the record and say that.

Take my grandfather. On Christmas Day, he was admitted to hospital, delirious, with a urinary tract infection. He was briefly treated and discharged back to the low-care facility he lived in. When I went to see him, he was confused, hot, sweaty, and rolling around in agony. The urinary tract infection was probably in his blood. It was affecting his mental state. And on examining him, it was obvious he also had a fractured hip. So here you have a 97-year-old, transferred back to hospital because of a urinary tract infection, with an untreated broken hip. From this point the likelihood that he can survive the infection, or a highly probable pneumonia or blood clot from lying in bed because of the broken hip, is very low. I subtly let my relatives know they should think about saying goodbye. But no, Grandad wasn't ready to die. He survived. I didn't use the stick, but as I have already said, it wouldn't have mattered that time round. He had the genetic resilience to survive.

But no matter what your genes are, they don't tell your full health story. You have the power to make good health choices and tip the scales in your favour. Look at it this way, a good decision can extend your life. A bad decision can get your balls caught in a plastic shower chair.

SUGAR

I can't think of anything on the planet that is more useless than soft drink—nipples on a man maybe—but other than that, nothing. Outside of pleasure: it tastes nice. I don't think there is anything wrong with treating yourself to something that tastes nice now and then. I do it all the time. But nutritionally speaking, soft drink is useless. There are plenty of other examples of modern day food products that are filled with sugar and not much else, confectionery is a good example. I guess my major issue with soft drink is that it's such an easy way to consume huge amounts of empty, useless calories. You don't even need to expend any energy chewing, like you have to with a donut. Just grab a two-litre flagon of your favourite poison, a funnel, open your gullet and pour. Some talented people don't even need to swallow. (Pretty sure I may have just ruined any chance of scoring a soft drink endorsement deal.)

Sugar is everywhere, not just in soft drink. There is the sugar you know about; the obvious stuff. Then there's the not-so-obvious sources. This makes cutting out sugar very tricky. And if you've decided that's an adjustment that you want to make in your diet get ready for the challenges, and be realistic about how hard it will be initially. But I think it's important we all try to cut back on sugar, especially the obvious stuff.

The average person shovels in 300 calories from added sugar every day, according to a recent report from the University of North Carolina. To put that in perspective, that's the equivalent of eating an extra 30,000 Skittles every year on top of all the other calories. I do love Skittles, but that's a bit excessive.

So, what can you expect if you cut out the sweet stuff?

If you've deciding to cut out sugar, be careful about setting yourself up to fail. You certainly will. Even the most dedicated humans on the planet fail. Don't beat yourself up. You are human and you will have bad days. You'll crave something that you've told yourself you are never going to eat. Your choice is to go ahead and eat the donut or drink the can of Coke or spend the entire day stressed out of your brain.

Would a sugar tax help? Do we need one? Do we want to live in a nanny state that makes decisions for us, that holds people's hands and makes them eat a certain amount of vegetables and fruit?

As I've already banged on about, the issue for me is that the information consumers are given is so tainted that a lot of times it's nearly impossible to make the right choice.

If I could trust the packaging and advertising of food products, fine. But I can't. I'm not saying that companies are out to intentionally harm you, but they're driven by profit, they're driven by the desire to sell product. They might tell you that something is 99% fat free. You buy the product because you're trying to make a healthy choice for yourself. If the company fails to disclose that after taking 99% of the fat out they added a lot more sugar, I think that that's a problem.

We've still got a way to go, but I think people have a better understanding of healthy living. As a doctor, I no longer feel that I have to give patients a list of the foods that they should eat and a list of foods that they shouldn't. You shouldn't smoke this and you shouldn't do that. I think that would be underestimating their intelligence. For whatever reason, there are some people who don't know the difference, but I think they're the exception. People know that a drive-through restaurant is going to be less healthy for them than eating fresh fruit and vegetables.

SET YOURSELF UP TO SUCCEED

Us humans respond to positive feedback. We love it. It's part of our make-up and gives us that nice warm, fuzzy feeling that makes us keep trying to reach our goal. Like most animals, I guess. If you set yourself up to succeed, with small incremental goals that you are more likely to reach, you set yourself up to thrive off the positive feedback, and before you know it you've reached your bigger goals. If you set yourself up to fail, with just large, long-term, challenging goals, then you don't get the benefit of having little positive boosts along the way. One little miss, the negative feedback kicks in and stopping yourself from quitting becomes really hard.

Think of achieving your health goals, and especially your eating goals, as a long flight of stairs. At the top of the stairs is ultimately where you want to be. It might be a goal weight, it might be a distance you want to run, it might be only eating one block of chocolate a month not one a day. Whatever that health goal is, visualise that as the top of the stairs. Then see every step as a new goal that you will need to reach along the way. Each goal should take you just a little bit closer to the top of the stairs. Start with half a block a day for the first two weeks. Then make a block last three days. Then make it last a week, then a week and a half. Two weeks. Three weeks and then you will be at the top of the stairs.

Don't get caught up in worrying about how many stairs, or little goals there are in your flight. If it's longer it might just work in your favour. Now I'm not giving you a licence to take forever, just don't be afraid to take your time—there is a very good reason why.

True success in health is when you don't have to think about being healthy. When being healthy is automatic, habitual. So, our health goals should really be the health habits we want. Given it takes 50–75 days to form a habit, depending on the research you read. There are lots of things working against you when it comes to creating healthy habits and turning unhealthy ones around, your mind, how your body adapts, other commitments, just life really, so don't be afraid to take the time required to work at it.

Alcoholics set themselves the goal of going one day

without alcohol. Then two. Then Three. Four. And so on. Feeling validated at the beginning of every new day that they have reached their 24-hour goal, helps fuel them with the positive feedback required to get through just one more day. And over time their body changes, it adapts and the ability to get through another 24 hours without a drink gets easier. Often there are stumbles along the way. Like there are for all of us. We are human after all.

When it comes to changing your diet, adding good foods need to be approached in the same way as cutting out the bad ones. One step at a time. Don't put yourself under the pressure of eating the perfect diet tomorrow. We've all been there. Lying in bed, staring at the ceiling trying to count how many calories are in a frozen ham and pineapple pizza, a bottle of wine, a bag of lolly snakes and a roll of cookie dough, vowing that tomorrow the perfect diet starts. And come 6 pm the next night you're talking into a drive-through speaker thinking tomorrow, yep tomorrow, the perfect diet starts tomorrow. Stop the cycle. There is no perfect diet. Small goals, positive feedback, and give yourself a break. Tomorrow try not to eat an entire block of chocolate and you're off and running.

Let's say you'll live to 85. Do you think the next six weeks are going to change that much? What will change things, is deciding that for the next 50 years you're going to eat a commonsense diet that is palatable and nutritious. You are going to consume as little as possible of the things you shouldn't eat—all the sugars, processed meat, complex carbs. Here's a simple idea: start with avoiding things that come wrapped in plastic. Stuff doesn't get pulled out of the ground or fall from trees wrapped in plastic.

Cook more meals, eat a large breakfast focusing on foods that will fill you for the day. Proteins in eggs, good fats in avocado, whole grains. Eating a small breakfast and a large dinner is the wrong way round. Eat a breakfast that keeps you full longer and sets you up for the day. Try not to eat too much at night.

EDUCATE YOURSELF

We are all born ignorant, but one must work hard to remain stupid.

Benjamin Franklin

Self-education is important. It's impossible to know everything about health, no matter what the 'gurus' that are selling you something believe they have figured out. It's not about having all the answers, it's about teaching yourself how to find the right answers. Nutritional information on food packaging is tricky—that may turn out to be the biggest understatement in this book. A panel of hieroglyphics scratched onto the back of a postage stamp would be easier to decipher. Figures, and measurements and words that make sure the manufacturer satisfies some outdated disclosure requirement, that mean nothing for any of us trying to decide what is the right food for me and the family. Let alone the ever-creative marketing slogans. 'Reduced Salt'. 'Natural Ingredients'. '99% less fat' is my favourite. Less fat than what? The fat content of a tub of fat is 100% fat.

So, if I have 99% less fat than a tub of fat. I think I may still have too much fat. Yeah?

Making dietary decisions is treacherous every day. Not only for ourselves but also for our kids. It's nerve-racking. Trust me when I say the you are not alone during the morning ritual of staring into a mostly empty fridge deciding whether it's parental neglect to send your kids to school with a half-eaten wheel of camembert and some rich crackers for lunch. It's happening all over the world. Trouble is it's no joke. Kids learn their future eating habits from us as parents. Setting a good example, and educating our kids, is more important now than ever before.

During the past 40 years global rates of overweight and obese people have risen dramatically. In 2010, more than 155 million children worldwide were overweight (more than one in 10). Of these, between 30 million and 45 million were obese—that amounts to between two and three per cent of the world's 5 to 17-year-old children.

If you're cooking at home you are already doing well. Simply prepared fresh foods are the best. Cooking at home is an excellent time to get your kids involved with handling food, learning about food, tasting different foods and enjoying fresh unprocessed produce.

Would it be nice to be able to avoid all the foods that you know are bad for you? Have the 'perfect' diet? Sure. Does it increase your chance of avoiding a lot of lifestyle related disease? Yes, it does. Is it realistic? No. Bad foods taste nice. It's a fact. That's kind of the point. Highly processed, convenient foods, whether it's takeaway of pre-packaged, are produced to make us want more. And the more you eat the harder it is to not go back for more. Your reward centre is triggered, you feel good. So, you want to feel that again. You eat more. Understanding this is important.

I can't prescribe you the perfect diet. That would be slightly hypocritical of me. What I can do is tell you the general rules I think we should all apply when it comes to creating our own perfect non-perfect diet.

Tip one, it should be as much of the stuff we know we should eat as possible. How do you recognise what those things are? First tip, go for the things that humans haven't screwed around with too much. Fresh, unprocessed produce the way it fell from the trees or was pulled from the ground. There are no apple trees that have little snack packs with a friendly, smiley apple guy printed on them, hanging from their branches.

Tip two, colour, lots and lots of colour. Vegetables of all variety of colours must be the pillar of any diet. The more colourful your meals the more essential vitamins and minerals that you are eating. Sure, there are plenty of multivitamin pills you could buy, but none of them are as good as a colourful plate full of vegetables. If you consistently look at your plate and the dominant colour is brown, then you are not on the right track. Less brown, more orange, and green, and red, and purple and yellow. Just so I am being 100 per cent clear with this 'colour' point, let's do a quick quiz. What colour is carrot? Orange—filled with fat-soluble nutrient, vitamin A. It helps your body form healthy teeth, bones, soft tissues, and skin. It can also help you ward off bacterial and viral infections, prevent night blindness, and keep your hair and nails healthy.

What colour are hot chips? Brown—deep-fried in trans fats, significantly increasing your risk of cardiovascular disease including a heart attack or stroke.

What colour is capsicum? Green, red and yellow—jammed with vitamin C, also known as ascorbic acid. It's a powerful antioxidant that helps protect the health of your cells. It improves your body's iron absorption. It's also important for promoting healthy teeth and gums, healing wounds, and helping you resist infection.

What colour is a pie? Brown—it's filled with god knows what.

What colour is spinach? Green—provides vitamin K, which is critical for your body's formation of blood clots. Without it, you could bleed to death from a simple cut. It may also help maintain bone strength in older adults.

What colour is a donut? Brown—filled with cream and sugar and jam and saturated fat and icing and sugar.

I think I made my point. Also, for all you clever guys who put sauce and mustard on your pie and chips, and eat donuts, maybe, that doesn't count as adding red or yellow.

Tip three, commonsense. It's a solid tip for all health decisions, but especially when it comes to food choices. A packet of chips once a month is not going to kill you. A packet of chips every day is tipping the scales. Western society is obesogenic, that means it tends to make avoiding obesity harder. Our world is overweight. Once that would have been an outrageous statement. But now it's a fact. And the World Health Organization backs it up with stats:

- Worldwide obesity has more than doubled since 1980.
- In 2014, more than 1.9 billion adults, 18 years and older, were overweight. Of these over 600 million were obese.
- 39% of adults aged 18 years and over were overweight in 2014, and 13% were obese.
- Most of the world's population live in countries where overweight and obesity kills more people than underweight.
- 41 million children under the age of five were overweight or obese in 2014.

We have to accept these facts. It's not about pointing the finger or shaming anyone, those are the cold, hard statistical facts. Those stats are the result of the world we have created. Food that is high in energy. That is, the food that we eat, that then gets converted by our bodies into stored energy, otherwise known as fat, is the easiest to get, the most heavily marketed and in a lot of cases the cheapest.

A lot of people are very busy. We have jobs, families, and try to squeeze exercise into what little time we have spare. Twenty-five years ago, we weren't eating takeaway seven nights a week, or high-energy foods all day. And we were much more active.

We have made our bed and now we have to lie in it. Or do we?

You aren't going to change that world right away but you can change the way you live in it. You don't have to tolerate it. You can make decisions that mean you exist in a much healthier way.

What is your relationship with food? Do you spend most of your time thinking about your next meal? Do you find that you can't wait for lunch or afternoon tea? Is food the first thing you think of when you get home? On most days my answers to the above questions will be complicated.

I'm not a huge fan of the 'relationship' with food statement, because I think a lot of us use it as an excuse, and for most it's complicated. Everybody has a relationship with food. In the same way that everyone has a relationship with air. You need it. It's in your life. You have to deal with it every day. Therefore, you have a 'relationship' with it. The important part is how you deal with food in your life. Is it just a source of energy to live your life? Is it all you think about? Do you rely on it for comfort? Do you avoid it? Does it bring you joy? Does it bring you anguish?

It's important to understand these are questions you need to be able to answer honestly—like with any relationship—to understand how you can create a 'healthy' relationship with food that works for you. Keep in mind your 'relationship' with food, may be a specific issue you have with food, or it might be a symptom of something else that you have an issue with. I will talk more about relationship and mental wellness later in the book, but what I will say now is that the first step is recognition. First understand the role food has in your life, and if it isn't as good as it could be, recognise that and then you can start doing something about it.

The problem for a lot of people is that food preparation is hard. I love to cook. But I'm far from the world's greatest

MasterChef. I've got my 'go-to' meals that I have been wheeling out for years. I add to the repertoire now and then, but most of the time it's about doing the things I am most comfortable doing, and creating 'wanky' names to makes myself seem more accomplished than I am. Isn't that what all chefs do? My crispy hand-raised molly-coddled chicken breast, wrapped in quadruple-smoked, wafer-sliced prosciutto stuffed with foraged forest mushrooms and locally harvested micro greens, is a real classic.

Jokes aside, if you are not a fabulous cook, the evening dinner question of 'What am I going to cook for the family?' can end up leaving your feeling more stressed and the glass of wine you just poured getting filled up again pretty quickly.

You want to remove as many moments of stress and 'fear of failure' as possible. Start by thinking about what you are going to eat. That's easier. Have food in your fridge and cupboards that you like to eat, that is easy to prepare and that you are happy to eat consistently. For me that means really simple things to cook that I enjoy: lots of eggs, chicken, tuna, vegetables that taste nice raw and in salads. Red meats now and then but not so much.

Don't be afraid to make things that you can cook consistently. Eat meals that make you feel good. If you have a big heavy pasta meal and it makes you feel like rubbish, then don't eat it.

Avoid heavily refined cereals with sugar and milk for breakfast—you are setting yourself up to crash later in the day. What is going to make me feel good in the morning? Whip a couple of eggs in a bowl and throw them in the microwave, grab an avocado, a slice of wholegrain toast and you're set.

And remember, the way you eat is the way your kids will eat. They learn how to walk and talk by watching all that you do. Trust me, they are watching. I figured this out one day when I was driving in traffic and a guy made an illegal right-hand turn right in front of me. I slammed on the brakes, hit the horn as hard as I could and before I could get the word out of my mouth I heard from the back seat 'Dickhead'. My three-year-old son had definitely been paying attention.

THE REALITY CHECKUP

Q: How important in portion control in my diet?

AR: Hugely important. Modern processed foods are jammed with energy which means most of the time we are taking in more calories than we need. Add to that the fact that the size of a standard meal has also increased. A quick way to counteract that is reduce the size of the meal. Just eat half as much. Split meals instead of eating them all yourself. Eat off bread plates instead of dinner plates. Challenge yourself not to finish an entire meal. Any way of reducing the amount you eat will help. Throw in better food choices and you will definitely tip the scales in your favour.

Q: What is the ideal breakfast for a busy day?

AR: There is no perfect answer but I love eggs. Lots and lots of eggs. Avocado. Wholegrain toast. Tomatoes. Protein is good. 'Good fats' are good too. Foods that fill you up. It doesn't have to be gourmet, just tasty enough that you'll be excited about eating it again tomorrow.

Q: If there is one thing I could cut out of my diet to improve my overall health, what would it be?

AR: You can answer this one. Be honest with yourself. If you take a moment to run through your regular diet I'm sure you can think of one thing, maybe two, and if you're like me, there is actually a laundry list to choose from! It will most likely be that thing you love most, that you feel guilty after eating and is your 'go to' choice when you need a food pick-me-up. It might be refined sugars, processed carbs (such as white breads and pastas), alcohol, pastries, soft drinks, pies or burgers, but whatever it is start simple, set realistic goals and build on your success.

Q: How import is what I eat for other members of my family?
AR: Unless your kid is significantly advanced—a food prodigy perhaps who can shop and cook for the entire family—they will eat what you provide for them. They will also make food choices based on what you teach them. Good choices *and* bad choices. The nutrition of your kids is your responsibility until they are old enough to forage and hunt for themselves. Research also shows that the nutritional habits are formed in early life and are carried through to adulthood. So, by setting a good example you not only help them while they are young, you are also helping them when they finally leave home.

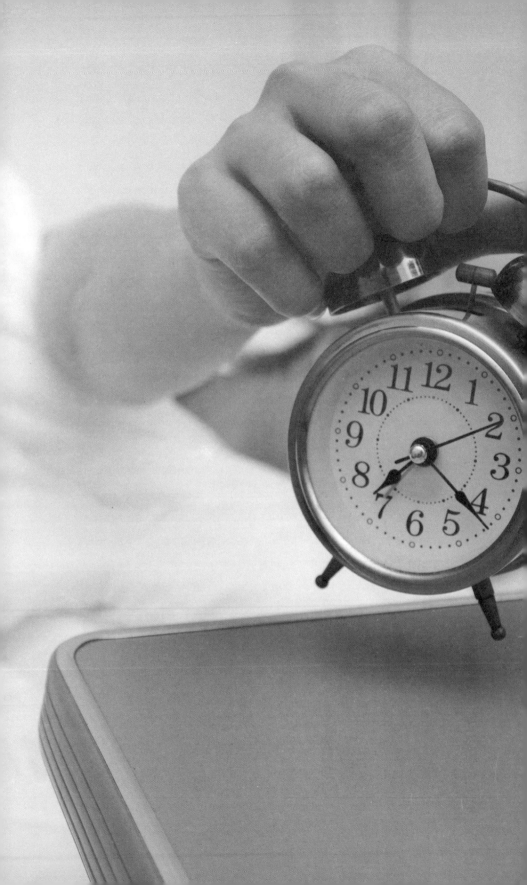

4. SLEEP

Sleep is that golden chain that ties health and our bodies together.

Thomas Dekker

I will happily go on record to say that sleep is the most underrated element of the modern obsession with being as healthy as possible. We constantly hear about the latest diet, or exercise regime, but rarely do we hear about how important sleep is.

How important is sleep? Well, let me put it this way. Not sleeping will kill you faster than not eating. To put it another way. Sleep deprivation is deadlier than starvation. Don't ask me who signed up for the research study that figured that out, but you get the point that sleep is important.

What can you do to maximise your potential for a perfect night's sleep? Well, firstly let's find out what kind of sleeper you are. And what better way to do that than to use history's influential overachievers and their infamous sleeping patterns. Are you a Da Vinci? A Kennedy? Or a Bonaparte?

About one to three per cent of the population are 'short sleepers' and these people need less than the recommended minimum of six hours of sleep per night. It appears they have an advantage that most of us don't have. According to researchers, they are blessed with a gene variant that allows them to go about their daily tasks normally after much less sleep than is generally recommended.

Former British Prime Minister Margaret Thatcher, successful businesswoman Martha Stewart and President Donald Trump, all claim to have regularly had, or still only need, three to four hours sleep a night. Renowned inventor and electrical engineer Nikola Tesla gained notoriety as a 'mad scientist' for his unusual sleep patterns. He claimed that he rarely slept more than two hours a day and reportedly once worked 84 hours in his laboratory without sleep.

Then there are the sporadic sleepers. Like Napoleon Bonaparte. When at war, Napoleon was a model of energy for his soldiers, fighting alongside his troops and developing war strategy for days on end. The emperor seldom changed his clothes or slept through the entire night and was known for his ability to nap. Though an insomniac during times of stress, he occasionally managed to catch up on his sleep: after campaigning, he was rumoured to sleep for at least 18 hours straight.

Leonardo Da Vinci excelled in multiple genres—he was a painter, sculptor, architect, engineer, inventor, mathematician—but sleeping wasn't something he had mastered. He famously tended to leave products unfinished.

Some believe this could be attributed to his sporadic sleep schedule, which consisted of taking short naps throughout the day instead of ever sleeping at night.

Or maybe you're more of a napper? After a mid-morning stint of swimming and exercise, John F Kennedy would eat his lunch in bed and then settle down for a nap. He would have his valet draw the drapes and ask not to be disturbed unless it was a true emergency. He would then quickly fall asleep for a one-to-two-hour nap. Jackie would always join him no matter what she was doing when her husband's nap commenced, leaving an assistant to entertain her guests. Head of the household staff, JB West, recalled that 'during those hours the Kennedy doors were closed. No telephone calls were allowed, no folders sent up, no interruptions from the staff. Nobody went upstairs, for any reason.' Jackie was the one who later encouraged LBJ to take naps, telling him, 'It changed Jack's whole life.'

Winston Churchill was a devout napper saying, 'Nature has not intended mankind to work from eight in the morning until midnight without the refreshment of blessed oblivion which, even if it only lasts twenty minutes, is sufficient to renew all the vital forces'. A nap was so sacrosanct to Churchill that he kept a bed in the House of Parliament and believed that napping was the key to his success leading the country through the Battle of Britain.

Thomas Edison was something of a self-hating napper. He liked to boast about how hard he worked, how he slept only three or four hours a night, and how he would sometimes work for 72 hours straight. But in truth the key to his spectacular productivity was something he was loathe to mention and hid from others: daily napping. Once when his friend Henry Ford paid a visit to his lab, Edison's assistant stopped him from going into the inventor's office because Edison was snoozing. Ford said, 'But I thought Edison didn't sleep very much.' To which the assistant answered, 'He doesn't sleep very much at all, he just naps a lot.'

No matter their genetic make-up or personal preference the common theme is all these overachievers required quality sleep. And the same goes for us. Quality is most important, then quantity and then schedule.

For most of us the prescribed average is eight hours a night. There is no perfect formula for achieving those eight hours sleep but we can go a long way towards setting ourselves up for the necessary rest we need.

Lack of proper rest affects your daily performance—and your relationships. You don't feel good in yourself. If you're grumpy and irritable, there is a very good chance that lack of sleep will be the cause. However, there is one point that must be remembered. The older you get the less sleep you'll need. It might be because age has slowed you down during the day and your body doesn't need a full eight hours sleep, but scientists have also found in a new study that a cluster of neurons associated with regulating sleep patterns might die off as we get older. In many cases, by the time people have reached the age of 70 and beyond they sleep for only six or six-and-a-half hours. The downside of this is that they don't feel as rested the next morning—they just haven't been able to sleep for any longer.

I recommend those eight hours and on a regular basis. You can't go into what I would describe as sleep debt. You can't bank sleep. By that I mean you can't sleep for 10 hours one night and then tell yourself that you can lose two hours the following night, having only six hours sleep, because you had those extra hours the night before. However, if you break from your pattern of eight hours every night and then suddenly have only six hours one night, you can make up for it by sleeping for 10 hours the following night.

A regular routine is vital. Try not to vary your sleep patterns. Go with your body's flow, what I would describe as 'sleep drive', setting yourself up for that perfect night's sleep later.

ENGAGING YOUR SLEEP DRIVE

What you do during the day determines how you get your sleep drive into gear to lead you towards a good night later. Obviously, the passage of time increases the sleep drive, but various activities (even exercising, if you have the opportunity) will add to the drive to sleep, along with the body's natural rhythm.

It's natural for our bodies to sleep when it is dark and be awake when it is light, so as the daylight hours slip by our bodies tell us that we are heading towards the sleep zone. What is beginning to come into play here is a natural hormone called melatonin, which is produced by the pea-sized pineal gland found just above the middle of the brain. This gland is asleep during the day when we're up and about, working, playing and exercising. But, like flicking on an electric light switch, the gland turns itself on and begins to produce melatonin as the end of the day approaches. Darkness stimulates melatonin and melatonin makes you sleepy. An average time for this to occur is around 9 pm. As melatonin levels in the blood continue to rise, we begin to feel sleepier, less alert. I know what you're thinking, 'but my favourite discotheque (who knew that's how you spell it!) doesn't start pumping till at least 9 pm!' Sorry, that doesn't stop melatonin telling us it's dark and we should be thinking of sleeping, it just means you put it off a bit longer while you get jiggy with it.

We might be able to get away with very late-night activities for a few nights but unless we start on a pattern of night-shift work, when we reverse our body's sleep expectations and form a false night in a darkened room during daylight hours, prolonged deprivation of sleep will have a detrimental effect. The melatonin effect shouldn't be ignored. As an example, researchers who studied the use of melatonin as a sleeping tablet found that people got to sleep some seven minutes quicker than normal and stayed asleep for eight minutes longer. They also improved the quality of their sleep (not that I am advocating a tablet form of what occurs naturally).

STRATEGIES FOR SLEEP

You have to give yourself down time before going to bed, getting rid of stress, for example, because worry keeps the mind ticking over. An active mind is the scourge of a good night's sleep.

There are tricks you can pull to slow down the mind and one that I've tried myself is to write down all your worries or unfinished tasks, if you have any, and send them in an email to yourself. If you prefer, write them down on paper, setting them aside to be attended to the following day. I can guarantee you won't be solving all the world's problems that night so best to be rid of them for at least eight hours. Send them to another place, lock them away in the computer or in that notebook and tell yourself that's all done for the day. This will help to get yourself into a routine of heading to a place where you are relaxed away from the concerns of the day that has gone by, preparing yourself for the one that is soon to arrive.

Another trick. As the time for bed approaches, or even when you're in bed and unable to sleep, take yourself in your mind to a far-flung corner of the world, to a long beach where you might be enjoying a gentle snooze in a hammock, to the sound of the gentle lapping of the tide flowing in from a turquoise sea. In other words, let your mind send you off on holiday. Above all, getting into bed should be your way of finding refuge from all the worries of the day. Good health will go a long way towards achieving that relief because it does help to put you into a relaxed state of mind.

The brain is made up of electrical components that are on the go all the time. Your body might be lying still in bed but your brain continues to do a lot of thinking for you. It might create a situation in your mind where you are running from danger, or it's dragging you back into the problems of the previous day. There's a danger of putting your brain in a tough spot, something like being between a rock and a hard place. You want your brain to solve the world's problems but at the same time you're wishing it could help you relax and get to sleep.

By pushing your brain when you're trying to sleep you're forcing yourself to stay awake and when the new day starts your problems are still there. It's like a football player—no point in pushing to the edge of exhaustion when it's only a practice match. Your brain does a lot of housekeeping when you're resting, silently droning on without the need for you to join in, forcing it to do more.

If you want evidence that your brain is still working when, hopefully, you're fast asleep, then dreams should make that pretty clear. It creates dreams for you and there's every chance that if you're in a relaxed, happy, state of mind when you drop off you'll have pleasant dreams. The bad dreams come when your thoughts are in turmoil after an unhappy day. And if you have nightmares, perhaps that's just your brain being cruel.

WHAT ELSE?

What then, aside from you refusing to let go of problems that surround you, are the other elements that impact on sleep? What comes to mind immediately is alcohol. Be honest, who's poured themselves a large glass—or three— of something at the end of a long day in the hope it will ensure a good night sleep? There's no doubt that it's an inducer of sleep. Think of the image of the man who's had more than enough and is slumped over, fast asleep on the bar. Alcohol depresses the central nervous system, your brain, and large amounts of it will certainly put you into old sleepy land, but it certainly doesn't help you to have quality sleep. You tumble out of bed the following day feeling like you haven't slept a wink because, although you don't remember spending the whole night awake, you certainly didn't get the sleep you needed. Alcohol prevents you from reaching the stages of sleep that you need every night to feel rejuvenated. So, the entire night is spent in a light slumber, not a quality one.

And there's coffee and tea, both stimulants. If you drink either of those close to bedtime there is a chance you'll find sleep difficult. It's the same with large meals late at night. Let's forget about those European countries that don't eat dinner 'til midnight. One reason they are able to slip into a good sleep is that they've been eating late all their lives and their bodies are used to midnight dining. For most of us, big meals late at night leave us feeling awkwardly full with an elevated metabolic rate as our inside struggles to churn, shift and digest a gut full of food.

Too hot in bed? And I'm not talking naughty 'hot', I'm talking temperature, uncomfortable, kick the covers off and don't touch me kind of hot. Your body needs to cool to be able to fall asleep, so if you feel the way I just described, it is almost impossible to fall asleep. Do whatever you can to cool down. Nude up, crank the fans, open windows, cool wet towels, hang your leg out of the bed, whatever works. In those situations, getting your body to cool is the key, but believe me, I know it's a lot easier than it sounds.

One trick to use the body-heat factor in your sleeping favour, which may seem counterintuitive to start with, is to have a hot shower before going to bed. Yes, hot, not warm or cold. Hot. After you have artificially raised your body temperature with a hot shower, your body temperature will begin to drop back to normal, creating the same physiological effect as when your body temperature drops during cooling.

Just as a quick aside, don't overdo the 'cooling down', getting to sleep when you're cold can be as difficult as sleeping when you're too hot.

In this high-tech age, we live on our computers, tablets and smartphones. They're in cafes, all forms of transport, the living room, the kitchen, the bathroom (I know you check your phone on the toilet, or is that just me?) and in the bedroom. Yep, we love our electronics in the bedroom. This isn't necessarily the best idea, especially if you are already having trouble sleeping. Taking an electronic device to bed, perhaps to watch a movie on a tablet or catch up with some work on a laptop, is a brain stimulator and if you've been taking in my earlier advice you'll know what that means.

Admittedly, everybody is different. I was talking to someone recently who finds the best way he can get to sleep is to pop in an earpiece, so he doesn't disturb his partner, and listen to the radio. He drops off to sleep in minutes and even though the late night chat shows are playing all night through the earpiece he wakes up feeling fine, because he's found his way of enjoying that vital eight hours.

At daybreak, we begin the process towards sleep; it's an inevitability. What you do from that moment on will affect how you sleep that night. A bright sunny start with a good healthy breakfast will set you up and by 2 pm you are at your peak. But sometime later, perhaps around 3 pm, especially after a heavy lunch, there is a very good chance you will start to feel sleepy. That's because of something called our circadian rhythm—our natural body clock. It has two peaks during a 24-hour cycle, 3 am and 3 pm. That mid-afternoon slump, when you're sitting at your desk staring at your computer reading the sentence 12 times craving a carb-loaded snack, is a dead giveaway. The quick fix of an afternoon energy drink and a bag of sherbies will work in the short term, but makes things worse in about an hour.

Go with a solution that sustains you through to bedtime. Exercise around 3 pm can work for some. Foods like nuts are better than sweets. Or maybe we should follow the lead of Kennedy, Churchill, Portugal, Spain, the Philippines, Malta and much of Latin America by having an afternoon siesta.

More than 85 per cent of mammalian species are polyphasic sleepers, meaning that they sleep for short periods throughout the day. Humans are part of the minority of monophasic sleepers, meaning that our days are divided into two distinct periods, one for sleep and one for wakefulness. It is not clear that this is the natural sleep pattern of humans. Young children and elderly people nap, and according the American National Sleep Foundation there are very clear health benefits from a short 20 to 40-minute lie down in the afternoon.

Naps have been shown to restore alertness, enhance performance, and reduce mistakes and accidents. A study at NASA on sleepy military pilots and astronauts found that a 40-minute nap improved performance by 34 per cent and alertness 100 per cent.

Daytime sleepiness, looking for the chance to have a nap at times other than associated with our natural body clock, along with irritability, is a sure sign that you aren't getting the sleep you need. Broken, restless sleep can also be a sign of health problems. Snoring—and 40 per cent of men and 30 per cent of women snore at some time—can be an indication of sinus problems, nasal polyps, obesity which increases fat tissue around the neck, and other threats to health. Worse, loud snoring can be a sign of sleep apnoea, which increases the risk of high blood pressure or even premature death. Sleeping partners are best placed to warn that things are wrong after listening to the person on the next pillow snoring loudly followed by significant pauses.

That's not good.

SNORING

One of the biggest reasons people don't sleep is that their partner wakes them up. Is your partner a snorer? A mover? A farter? Maybe you are. You have to think about what's the best way to get yourself a good night's sleep.

In a perfect world, which we know doesn't exist, you would probably sleep by yourself in soundproof, humidified, ventilated, dark, temperature-controlled room. But that's not reality. So, what's the perfect non-perfect sleep scenario?

I think it's one minimises the things that are most likely to keep you awake, and explores the best alternative for things that are not ideal. Sleeping alone isn't always by choice, but if you do have the opportunity, find a way to help resolve your partner's moving or snoring or farting, or whatever the disturbance is. It's important to explore whether you are genuinely being kept awake by your partner. Is there snoring that needs to be investigated? Are they moving around? Are they anxious?

I think exploring your problem from that point of view is better than trying to get yourself into a perfect sleeping space. Look at the imperfect and figure out how to manage it.

For a very long time, snoring was supposed to be something that only blokes did. You got to a certain age and you just snored. But the research and thinking changed and it's well established now that it's not normal. Being a noisy breather is not normal. There's research that shows that kids who snore are getting poor-quality sleep and it can affect their ability to learn. Understanding why someone is snoring is very important.

SLEEP APNOEA

As obesity becomes more of a problem the most common 'bedfellow' of snoring is sleep apnoea. There are two different types of sleep apnoea, but the one we're talking about is obstructive sleep apnoea. There are muscles that hold your airway open in the back of your throat and in your neck. During the day while you're awake, they're tense, neurons firing away to keep them working and contracted. They keep your airway open and that's a big part of the reason why you don't snore during the day.

When you fall asleep you go through different stages of sleep. You relax and the muscles that hold your airway open relax. For a lot of people this isn't a problem. If you don't have anything obstructing your airway, you won't snore. The air will still move as it's meant to and there will be no noise. But if you've got a lot of weight around your neck and around your upper chest, if you've got a big tongue or large adenoids and big tonsils, all those elements start encroaching on your airway. When you breathe in, the airway is smaller. The rest is physics. If air is moving through a floppy tube that's small, it vibrates and that makes a noise.

The problem with obstructive sleep apnoea is that it gets to the point where you're obstructing your airway so much that you can't breathe. If you've got somebody next to you in bed that does this, you'll know what I mean. Snore, snore, snore, big breath in—and then nothing. Still nothing. A bit more nothing. Then. Big gasp. Snore. Snore. And so on, all night. It sounds like they've stopped breathing, and it can seem like forever if you're lying there listening.

When you're snoring and you stop breathing the drive to breathe has to kick back in. The thing that drives us to breathe is carbon dioxide; we're not driven to breathe by oxygen levels, we're driven to breathe by rising carbon dioxide levels in the blood.

The carbon dioxide levels have to come up to a certain point before you gasp for air and take another breath. You wake yourself up just enough to open up your airway, but not enough to know you have woken up. That's why people with severe obstructive sleep apnoea who live alone can go for years without knowing anything is wrong They just spend their days never knowing why they are so tired and dreaming of a good night's sleep. If you're driving a truck or sitting at your desk, you feel like you haven't slept for days. And that's because you're not getting the quality sleep that you need. You're constantly being aroused.

People suffering from sleep apnoea have been studied in sleep clinics where their sleep is monitored. They're constantly being brought into a state of wakefulness the entire night, but the next morning they say their sleep was fine. They don't remember.

The science around obstructive sleep apnoea and quality of sleep is a pretty progressive part of medicine, in the scheme of the things. It hasn't been around for that long. We now have a better understanding of the risks of obstructive sleep apnoea: not getting a good night's sleep, being oxygen deprived at night and the impact of that on the brain, the risk of heart disease, the risk of stroke. And of course, the next day your risk of injury goes up because you're so fatigued.

If you snore it's important to know why. You might have a big tongue or big adenoids and they're not actually fully obstructing your airway—you're just a noisy sleeper. But if you're at that point where your airway is obstructed, that could have a huge impact on your health.

There are solutions. There are machines that people can use, you can lose weight, and a lot of other things, but the important part is the diagnosis. If the tell-tale signs are there—snoring, noisy breathing, stopping breathing and daytime fatigue—there is a very good chance you've got it.

You just haven't been told yet.

If your partner is having this discussion with you, you need to be listening because it's affecting their health—they're not sleeping properly either. Just as importantly, it's affecting your health too. You've got to respond. There's a solution—you have to go and get it.

THE REALITY CHECKUP

Q: What is the optimum amount of sleep I should try and get?
AR: There is no magic number but textbooks would say between seven and nine hours. Anyone who has had a young child is probably currently laughing those numbers. And I completely understand if you currently have a newborn that you have probably thrown the book across the room. I'm just repeating the science. At different times in your life you will get more, and then sadly there are the times you will get less.

Q: Should I be worried about my snoring?
AR: Snoring should never be something that is ignored. If you're the guy that people avoid sleeping in the same room with because you sound like a Boeing 747, that's not a good sign. There are plenty of reasons why you might be snoring, and there are also plenty of ways of reducing it so don't ignore it. And definitely don't ignore it if your sleeping buddy says that you stop breathing at any point, or you find that you wake up every day exhausted even though you think you have had a good night sleep. These are telltale signs you have a sleeping issue.

Q: What are the triggers for a bad night's sleep I should be aware of?
AR: Everyone has different triggers. When you figure out yours, do your best to avoid them. For some people its afternoon caffeine, others it's exercise that keeps them awake and for some its exercise that puts them to sleep. Alcohol can disrupt sleep, as can stress. Being too hot. Being too cold. Small, crying children too! Sorry,

that's not overly helpful, but all I can say is for bad sleepers there are usually a few things that make it worse. So, find your sleep saboteur and avoid it. Unless, of course, it is a small crying child. The good news is, they do grow up.

Q: What if it is my partner who is the 'sleep' problem?
AR: Get a new partner. Only joking. Tell them. Talk to them. Help them get it sorted. It will not only work for them it will also work for you. After that? Get a new partner.

Q: What is a good, pre-sleep ritual for getting a good night's sleep?
AR: If you're a bad sleeper, routine is a good place to start. Go to bed at the same time and get up at the same time every day. Yep, every day. Weekdays, weekends, days off, holidays. Routine and setting your internal body clock has a huge influence over sleep. Also have a wind down routine that sets you up for a good night's sleep. Have a shower. Read a book. Get rid of the electronics. When you find whatever it is that works for you stick with it. But don't overthink any of this. I know that's hard and I'm the guy telling you to think about it (I am aware of the irony) but don't overthink it. Overthinking about trying to sleep while you're trying to sleep will only make it impossible for you to sleep.

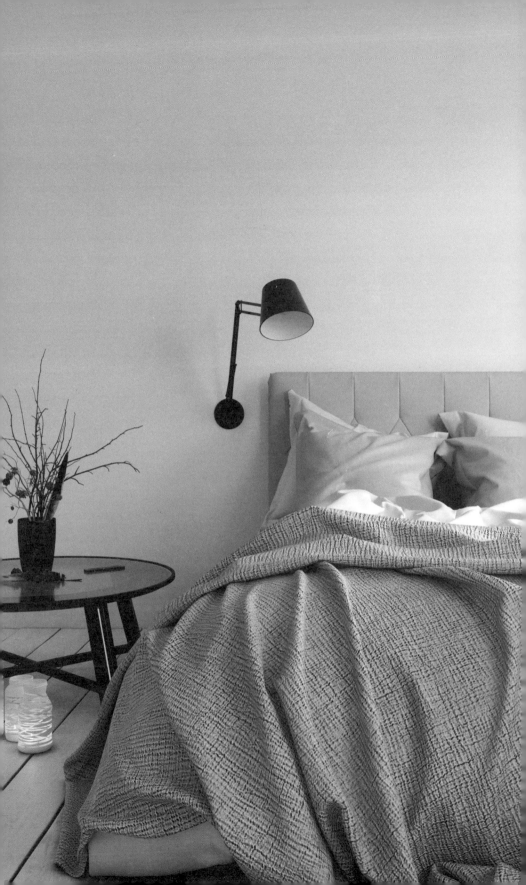

5. THE BEDROOM

Remember, sex is like a Chinese dinner. It ain't over 'til
you both get your cookie.

Alec Baldwin

I thought I'd kick things off with an understatement. Communication in the bedroom is important. Der. But so are a lot of other things. This chapter is about working through some of those important things. Am I an expert—a 'sexpert'—nope. So, I think it's best for me to stick to the things I know.

I know some stuff about anatomy. I know some stuff about physiology. I know some stuff about psychology. And I know enough about women to say that I don't know enough about women to claim to be any kind of bedroom expert. So, I'm going to stick to the bedroom health stuff—mainly for men.

There are a number of things that impact on sex. Most important is being in good physical condition. A healthy heart ensures that the toolkit is in good shape. It's actually the heart that plays a major role in ensuring that the penis is working well, because the heart is the pump that sends blood to the important vessels that make the penis erect. Think of the penis as a water balloon. That's not meant to be a statement about size as I am fully aware of the fact that water balloons are thoroughly unimpressive with regards to size. That's not to say if your penis is the size of a water balloon that I'm judging you; I'm not at all! I'm merely using an average-sized male appendage as my reference and it is larger than a water balloon. Anyway, blood makes a penis erect, rather like filling up a water balloon.

An out-of-condition heart means poorer circulation, less 'filling-pressure' and a penis that has a difficult time standing to attention. If you want to perform at your best in the bedroom your heart has to be kept in good shape—healthy heart, healthy water balloon.

On the food front, a good blood supply to the penis can be enhanced by a diet that includes avocados, vitamin B1, kidney beans and peanuts. It doesn't do any harm to eat onions, garlic, chili and, if you can take it, a good old Indian curry. These foods have been shown to improve the health of small blood vessels and improve blood flow to areas like fingertips, toes and the penis. Smoking has the opposite effect, it destroys small blood vessels, cutting off blood supply, especially to areas like fingers, toes and penis. We've all seen those old school movie scenes where lovers sit back in bed and light up a cigarette after sex, but whether anyone smokes before or after, it's not going to help the next time around.

One of the greatest concerns among men is size. Is it so important? Well I'm not the best judge of that, but maybe some keen researchers can help us figure it out. In a study conducted over a two-year period out of a Cairo Andrology Clinic, 92 men between the ages of 18 and 54 were examined. Their major complaint was that of a small penis, both flaccid and stretched. According to research the men understated the size of their penis. Okay. I can hear women all over the globe scoffing, but I'm just quoting the research. The study, published in the journal *Urology,* found that all 92 patients who complained of stunted penises actually had normal-sized members. Several even had longer-than-average endowments.

Slightly more than half of the men, 54 per cent, attributed their angst to childhood, when they began comparing their genitals to those of their friends. And 41 per cent said their concern began in adolescence, as they started watching erotic movies and reading pornographic magazines.

So, what is normal? A flaccid penis is considered normal if it is four or more centimetres and with the average being nine centimetres. The norm for an erect penis, where the appendage is measured from the tip, is seven or more centimetres, with an average of 13 centimetres.

The good, and perhaps rather surprising news, is that small penises increase in size more than a larger flaccid model. A penis may curve to the left, right or straight up. A curve is not necessarily a defect.

While I've never actually seen a broken penis, I have heard in recent times of a man in Vietnam who reported to a local hospital that his member had 'snapped' while he was trying an experimental sexual position. I'm happy to report on his behalf that he is now up and running again.

And while I've never had to deal with a case like that, I have seen priapism, an erect penis that won't return to its normal flaccid state. Believe me, you don't want to experience this, as it is extremely painful—agony in fact. The problem is caused when blood gets trapped in the erection chambers and while there is no obvious reason, it does affect men in cases of certain blood problems, like malaria. There have been other cases caused by the misuse of certain medical drugs, including those that are used to treat depression. Poisonous spider bites, carbon monoxide poisoning and the use of street drugs such as cocaine can also have a negative impact.

Good health leads to good sex and it works the other way too. Good sex has a positive impact on overall health. People who have regular 'feel-good' sex feel happier about themselves.

GOOD SEX

The concept of a perfect relationship, and the perfect sexual relationship, is really tricky. And in keeping with this book, perfect non-perfection is more likely than perfection. Everyone is so different and there isn't any rule book. A lot of us nowadays are trying to hold ourselves up to some level of perfection when it comes to sexual prowess, physical image, shape and size. Once again, if you try to be perfect that's not necessarily attainable. It can actually have a very negative effect in the bedroom.

This is a weird way to look at it, and most people would frown, but who's the most important person in the sexual relationship? I think it actually has to start with you, because confidence is the key. You have to be confident, and so many people nowadays have their confidence battered and feel less worthy because they don't measure up to some media-generated standard. If you're not confident, I think you lose out. Your partner loses out too, because your performance is nowhere near as good as it could be.

I think if you asked people of both sexes they'd agree that self-confidence is a very attractive thing. What does it mean to be self-confident without being self-absorbed? Yes, it can become negative. Narcissism is not very attractive. If you're at the point where you're only really pleasing yourself, that won't make for a healthy relationship. You can't be looking at a calendar crossing off how many times this week, how many times this month, how many times...

I think it comes down to the communication. For you, once a week might be fine. For your partner, it might not be fine. We all have different levels of sex drive; our hormones are very different.

Men and women are also very different when it comes to what drives bedroom activity. I think the cliché that men are less emotional, while women tend to need a little bit more emotional affection, is probably broadly accurate. The point is whether you're communicating enough to make sure that your needs and the needs of your partner are being met.

If it's all about what your partner wants, that's a problem too. Is there a happy middle ground somewhere there? Yes, sure. And if you are lucky enough to be in a place where you're in complete sync with your partner, well, good luck to you. If we are aiming to be the best non-perfect version of ourselves, that's what it would look like—a situation where both parties are satisfied with the sexual relationship. Everybody's happy.

Is that attainable? Not always. Everything changes, one day to the next. You have a good day at work, you have a bad day at work. You have different cycles, different hormones. You have different feelings about yourself, which are the result of so many different factors. These things can influence what happens in the bedroom.

There's a physical need for sexual contact, which is extremely important from a health point of view. Studies show that sex helps protect you from some of the cardiovascular and other types of diseases that are so common nowadays.

Having a healthy physical sexual relationship is an important thing for all humans to have. But that's not actually the whole story. There are emotional needs to be met on both sides. To hammer home the point, sex is a pretty boring thing to be doing by yourself. You have to look at how you get to a place where you feel you're satisfying yourself and satisfying your partner.

GETTING IN TOUCH WITH YOUR EMOTIONS

For many Australian males, being in touch with your emotions is not something that's easy—or even considered for more than a moment. I think the younger generation, my son's generation, are probably a lot better at it than my grandfather's generation.

I think the big issue for men is the level of vulnerability that you actually have to reveal. Men like to feel they are in control of their emotions, whether they are or not. Some think this is an evolutionary thing; that's a dated evolutionary-biology way of looking at things. The issue is how in touch are we with our emotions and the emotions of others. Are we willing to be vulnerable?

I think it's pretty hard to find a situation outside of the bedroom that puts you in a similar position of vulnerability. And I think that it's important for guys to understand how to be vulnerable and to be emotional—to delve into another part of the male psyche. That's not a bad thing; it's actually a very healthy thing. From a physical health point of view, ignoring how you feel about yourself and those around you, can be damaging to your physical and mental health. Because, invariably, that builds stress. Stress, we know, releases hormones, neurotransmitters and other signalling factors into the blood stream that raise your heart rate, raise your blood pressure and increase your risk of premature death. Apart from the physical impacts there are mental health impacts, sadly, issues that we're seeing increase every year. The statistics for males, especially young males, are scary.

It's important to be in touch with your emotional life. I'm not saying that you have to cry at the Labrador puppy on the toilet paper commercial, I'm saying it's important to allow yourself to be prepared to let other people into that emotional side of who you are. I suppose the question arises: how do you find a way to navigate through that, especially if it doesn't come naturally?

I think that if you are willing to give a little bit of yourself, invariably, you get somebody else willing to do the same. It's a really simple concept, and I think it's seen in everything, whenever you interact with anyone. People are more willing to open up and trust you if you open up and trust them. I think we might find value in setting aside all the ways that men most commonly talk about the bedroom: my prowess, my length and how long I last. All that stuff that makes us feel big and masculine and bang our chests. It is important to feel like 'men' but why not set that aside for just a moment? I think nowadays it's a bit of a dated way of looking at how men should be, or how men are, in the bedroom or in the world in general.

Trust me when I say I haven't mastered it. And there is nothing more embarrassing that being emotionally honest with someone who isn't in the same place. But it's part of looking after yourself. It's part of training yourself for when you really do need to ask for help, be vulnerable, and open up.

Being a man today is different from being a man 100 years ago. That's not a bad thing. It's just another part of the world and society that has evolved. Take chivalry—old-fashioned politeness—it hasn't disappeared, well I hope it hasn't, but it has evolved. Of course, the problem with chivalry in today's world is that it carries undertones of condescension. Women don't need you to open the door for them; they're quite capable of opening the door by themselves.

And I absolutely applaud that way of thinking. But that doesn't mean that you still can't care about those things. There are no defined roles for men and women anymore. There isn't that sort of black and white—I buy dinner, you look pretty—definition. And I think that that's a really important progression in our society. Men respecting women and women respecting men should be the norm in nightclubs, in boardrooms, bedrooms, everywhere.

Before you even get to the bedroom, it's also about quality communication. What are our expectations? What are our mutual expectations about the bedroom? There can be no assumption of marital rights or relationship rights or friends with benefits, or however you want to put it. Not that you want to be sitting with your partner discussing your sex life like a sales agreement—it doesn't happen like that—but there has to be a mutual understanding. Good communication, quality communication about the various facets of your relationship actually enhances what happens in the bedroom.

Whether you're in a relationship or not, whether you're trying to find a partner or you have one, I think that for men there is a huge amount to be gained if you're willing to be opened up slightly to the emotional part of who you are. You won't completely lose the masculine way you have of presenting yourself, but there are huge benefits. I think that when it comes to trying to be the best non-perfect version of yourself, if you're completely shut off to having any level of emotional connection with another person when it comes to the bedroom, you're missing out.

There are different stages of life where the whole bedroom relationship serves different purposes. You go through a stage where it's a purely physical thing and that's all you're looking for. It can be quite narcissistic. You shouldn't think it's not the same on the other side—women are just as interested in physical contact. And not every partner you're with is going to fall in love with you. But when it does come to having an emotional connection with someone—not just in the bedroom but in all facets of life—you get what you give.

If we're talking the best non-perfect version of yourself in the bedroom, it's important to understand the physical nature of what occurs in the bedroom. That sounds like a ridiculous thing to say, but I'm not talking about physical attraction, I'm talking about physical exertion. To perform at your best, you've actually got to be in some level of physical shape—the better physical shape that you're in, the better you will perform in the bedroom.

If you struggle to get out of bed in the morning and you're not exercising on any level I can guarantee you right now you're not performing at your best in the bedroom. Part of sex is the physical effort that's required. You would train to run a marathon, to swim a race or win a championship. The more you train, the better you are, and the better you're going to perform. In the same way, I'm not saying that you should be practising with someone else, but there is evidence to suggest practising by yourself might improve your performance. Yes, I'm talking about masturbation for those that aren't keeping up.

MAKING IT WORK

Don't try for perfect. Be yourself, be real. And don't expect your partner to be perfect either. Down the centuries people have tried to figure out the formula. There is no formula. It doesn't work like that. If you want to be the best possible version of yourself, if you want to be a confident sexual partner, you have to understand that this is about much more than body parts coming together. It's so much more than that. But as I said right back at the beginning of this chapter I'm not a 'sexpert'.

Some days, it'll be straightforward and simple and you'll know exactly what to do. You've connected with your partner and everything will be crystal clear to you. It's two people who understand each other. Great. Happy days.

But, there will also be times when you are completely out of your depth. You will find yourself thinking so many different things. Am I doing it right? What have I done wrong? Is this going to happen? Is that signal what I think that signal is? I'm not in mood. They're not in the mood? I really just want to sleep.

A lot of the time you're probably just adding more and more stress and pressure. When it comes to sexual performance, mental stress is the most common reason for a poor performance. So, you want to make sure you're clear in your own mind. You want to make sure that you're confident, that you're settled and relaxed.

Everybody's different. Some people have a handful of sexual partners in their life and some people have a small nation's worth. Everybody's different. Everybody's fumbling through it but some people are more willing to expose themselves fumbling through it than others.

Some guys bang their chest about the number of sexual partners they've had. That's a bit misguided. Everyone's different. You don't have to be like the guy next to you. If you're comfortable and you're happy and you've found something that pleases you, then that's what it takes for you. Somebody else may have different reasons and may be searching for something else.

SAFE SEX

If you look at the statistics, there has been a rise in certain STDs. During the Grim Reaper times, when the dangers of HIV and unsafe sex were widely publicised and there was sexual education around STDs, there was a drop off in all STDs.

Sexually transmitted diseases haven't disappeared, they are still an issue, still a problem. Safe sex is about protecting not only yourself but protecting others. An STD that doesn't cause you many issues and is cleared up with a short course of antibiotics might cause infertility in a female partner. Is that something you really want to be responsible for? If you're having multiple partners you can never be 100 per cent certain.

Pulling on my grumpy, finger wagging doctor hat for a minute, you need to make sure that you are practising safe sex and that you are smart about it. Obviously, there are other associated issues like unwanted pregnancies. So, stop for a minute and think. The best non-perfect version of you is not going to get an STD.

PORNOGRAPHY

The worldwide web has brought us many wondrous things. Supposedly 95 per cent of us at some point have typed a word into Google to see if we have spelt it right. One of those wondrous things is porn. Lots and lots and lots of porn. That does read like I have spent days trawling through the internet counting porn sites. Well I wouldn't say days. Porn is part of the world now, that has its upsides and downsides.

A growing area of research suggests that what people are seeing on the internet could be creating a warped view of what sex is and how it should be performed and what relationships should be like. Just like the poor Egyptian guys in the study I mentioned at the start of the chapter, concerned about having small penises because of all the big ones swinging around the web. But it's actually not a far-fetched idea to think that kids nowadays won't be getting sex education from a book called *Where Did I Come From?* but from a couple of 'educators' called Cindy and Mindy.

I'm a parent, and I'm terrified access is so easy. In fact, the most advanced electronic device in our house is a cheese grater and it's not wi-fi enabled. Setting aside sending them to live with the Amish, I guess it's an extra area of communication that parents now have to navigate—the porn talk. Talking to them, however difficult that may be, will help them to a better understanding of human relationships.

It's a fact that the current generations enjoy a more open approach to sexuality. It's very different now but that's not necessarily a negative thing. However, it brings new challenges. Understanding those challenges and being willing to sit down, have the conversation, build those lines of communication with young people, is really important.

THE REALITY CHECKUP

Q: What health issues affect my performance in the bedroom?

AR: All. Yep, sorry to say it, but all aspects of health have an impact on how you perform in the bedroom—your diet, how fit you are, your mental well-being, your sleep patterns—everything. Think of yourself as a bedroom athlete. If you want to perform at an elite level then you have to train and get yourself into peak physical and mental condition. To achieve a gold medal, and the accolades that go with it, then it's going to take some effort. Lying around eating burgers dreaming of being an elite bedroom athlete will most likely lead to you competing against yourself. Where's the fun in that?

Q: How often should I have sex?

AR: A tricky one to answer because, unfortunately, you're not the only one involved in that decision, and there's no set rule or defined amount. At some stage in your life, you will undoubtedly have a friend who says they are having sex ten times a week but it's a moot subject. There's more to sex than frequency.

Q: How important is communication in the bedroom?

AR: Very. Talking to yourself doesn't count.

Q: Should I be concerned if I am losing my sex drive?

AR: Sex drive fluctuates over short cycles but also as we age. As hormone levels change so too does sex drive. But it's more about keeping it in perspective. Not wanting to have sex because you feel bad about yourself, or just don't 'feel' like it is different from a clinically significant fall in sex hormones leading to a genuinely abnormal sex drive. That said, if you have concerns it should be something that you feel comfortable discussing with your doctor, like all aspect of sexual health and wellbeing.

Q: What could be stopping me from having an erection?
AR: There are lots of physical and mental reasons why you might have difficulty getting an erection on any given day. The most common will be a psychological reason. Stress, anxiety, lack of self-confidence are major contributors to transient impotence. In most cases, if the cause of the stress or anxiety is resolved the engine room will go back to working. If it's a physical reason or persists, then further investigation may be required.

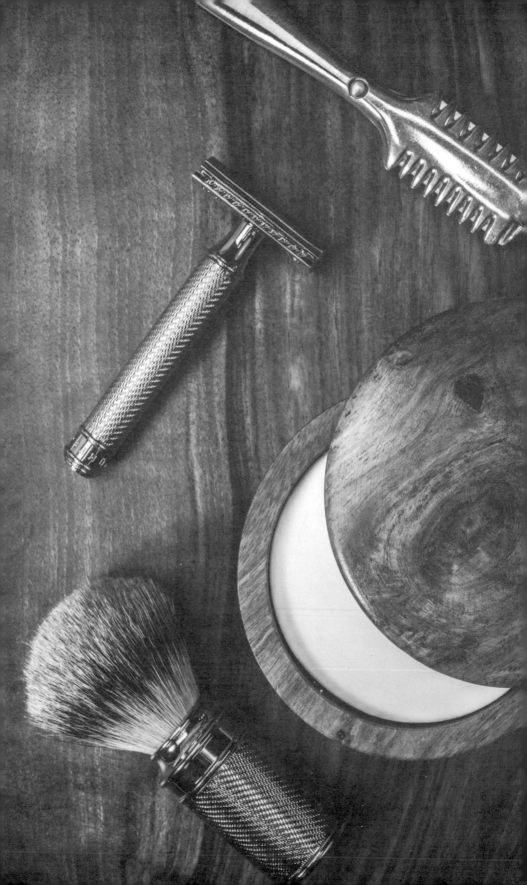

6. THE BATHROOM

Everything stinks till it's finished.

Dr Seuss

———

Try to set yourself up to follow a routine in the bathroom. It's not the military, so don't let it worry you, but routines and consistency can be good. For some of you, this will come naturally. For others, like me, there may be a little work involved.

Okay. You have a bowel movement, you urinate, shower, brush your teeth and, for those who don't want facial hair, shave. Was that too prescriptive? Are you a number one first number two second guy? Teeth then shower and shave fella? If I'm honest it doesn't matter, and everyone has their own pattern.

I'm going to go with the safest bet in the morning, and after a bit of a wait, usually what comes first is natural, starting at the toilet bowl. I don't intend to go into fine detail of what you should expect when you turn your early morning attention to that porcelain, but it will help to keep you at the top of your game to be aware of any problems that might be lurking. I don't want to send you out into the world if you aren't feeling up to scratch.

Urination is the emptying the body's liquid waste which, in this case, has built up while you slept. You might have paid a visit to the bathroom during the night as well, depending on whether you drank a glass of something before bedtime or you're driven there by the behaviour of your prostate.

CHECK OUT THE COLOUR

I've found that people are fascinated by the colour of their pee. Actually, it can tell you quite a lot about the state of your health. Urine has been an important part of diagnosis since the beginning of medicine. The colour, the smell and even the viscosity—by that I mean the thickness, you can have thick and thin urine—can tell doctors a great deal. At this point I need to add, I am not encouraging you to smell or measure the fluid mechanics of your morning wee. The key is paying attention to changes.

It may be that you've been eating a can of sardines, consumed asparagus, you're dehydrated, or you have a urinary tract infection—any of these factors can affect the colour. Most of the time the different colours you see are benign but if the urine is very dark over a long period or blood-tinged, it's time for a checkup.

So, you're standing over the toilet bowl and your flow is a pale straw colour. Perfect. Your health is good, you are well hydrated and you've earned yourself a high five. Find someone to celebrate with. Enjoy the moment. Then get back to business.

You don't want it to be paler or without colour at all, because that tends to suggest you're drinking too much water and it would be advisable to cut back. Water intake, and hydration tend to confuse people. There has been a long-held belief that you must drink eight glasses of water every day. Well that's a myth. It came about because the daily recommendation for an average-sized human is three litres of water. Health nuts in their eagerness not to read the fine print, interpreted this as three litres (about eight glasses) of water a day. Well if you do read the fine print it says three litres of fluid daily, including from all sources. Food, tea, coffee everything. So, the extra eight glasses of water actually tips you over the daily quota.

Okay, so we are happy that you're normal and healthy when you're hovering in the pale straw colour. Move a step up into a yellowish colour, but still transparent—also a good sign. After that, it pays to take heed of your pee's colour. A dark yellow is still recognised as being normal, but is a sign that you need to drink water soon.

Now, when it comes to the darker shades, it's time to be even more attentive. Honey-coloured urine is a sign that you should drink water immediately and if it's very dark or appears to have the consistency of syrup you are probably suffering from severe dehydration or worse, your liver might be diseased. I'd be concerned if you had time to stop and check your urine at this stage. Pink or a shade of red could mean you have blood in your urine. The good news is that this colour could also be the result of eating a vegetable or fruit with a red colour such as blueberries, beetroot or rhubarb. The bad news is that the reddish colour could be an indication of kidney disease, a tumour, a prostate problem or a urinary tract infection. Like with most things in health, go with the obvious answer first, and work through the likely causes from there. What that means is don't jump straight to bleeding prostate tumour if you've just eaten a beetroot burger with a side order of beetroot and a beetroot and rhubarb milkshake to wash it down. Okay?

Some men report a bubbly type of urine, sometimes looking like foam. This is often quite harmless—it's what is known as the hydraulic effect. I understand that makes your pipe sounds far more impressive than it may actually be, but it's actually just a way to describe the flow of urine. However, frothy urine could also suggest an excess of protein in the body or a kidney problem. Again, if this condition persists it's wise to check it out.

Here's some good advice, and not always top of mind when you're at the doctor's: at your next visit, for whatever reason, ask if you can have your urine tested, even if it's a normal colour. The reason for this is that sometimes blood in the urine, indicating a serious problem, is not visible to the naked eye. The laboratory checking your urine sample will also be able to establish the level of sugars in your body—an indication of whether you're at risk of diabetes.

So that's your urine. Self-diagnosis is fine up to a point, but if there's a persistence in that dark or pink colour, head to the doctor.

NUMBER TWO

While at the toilet bowl, it's a good time for me to pass on some guidelines about your poo. This is obviously not the most fascinating of topics (or perhaps it is!). Small children are fascinated by their poo. I've been told over and over again at most family gatherings that my favourite trick as a youngster was to use my toy lawnmower to mow it into the carpet of my bedroom. I should clarify that by youngster I mean two-year-old, not 15. I guess what I'm trying to say is you should have a healthy interest in your bowel movements, but not be using it for party tricks.

I can't judge what's going through your mind after you get up from the toilet seat, and I'm obviously not there with you—good news all round—but it might be worth my asking what your routine is. When you've finished your business, do you take a quick look before flushing it all away? My advice would be to do this from time to time to ensure everything is running normally.

The first question to ask is how regular are you? Surprisingly enough, the normal range is from a low end of three times a week right up to three times a day. That's a lot of leeway, so if you fall outside of these parameters, take it from me, there's a good chance something is awry, either with your diet or your body's plumbing. Lack of sleep, or stress, will also throw your bowel movements out of whack. You could be affected by travel into different time zones, failing to do adequate exercise, dehydrated or be suffering from fluctuating hormones. People who are regular can set their watch by the times they go. If you find yourself staring and pushing, groaning as you try to expel the waste, that's an abnormal amount of effort. If that sounds like you, I encourage you to think about what might be wrong. If that sounds like the guy in the cubicle next to you at work, I'll leave it up to you on whether you want to pass on your concern. Having a bowel motion should be as easy as peeing, but again, there can be typical or very unusual reasons for failing to be down and up from the toilet seat in a short time.

One of my patients came to me looking like he was pregnant. That's no joke. He had what could only be described as the gestational belly. I was pretty happy he wasn't pregnant, but something obviously wasn't right. On interrogation, he revealed the reason for him not pooing for more than a week was that he had eaten a four-kilogram bag of peanuts, and they were stuck. All of them. Right in his belly. A four-kilo peanut foetus! The correct term is bezoar—a mass of indigestible food that accumulates in the digestive tract and sets like concrete. The X-rays were not a pretty sight. He was facing two solutions, either being able to break down that nutty foundation stone in his stomach with drugs—softening him up—or resorting to surgery if that didn't work. Fortunately for him we were able to soften him up and he returned to a normal life, and most likely eating peanuts on the couch.

What then should you expect of your morning's deposit?

Healthy stool, as your poo is medically known, needs to be of medium to light brown colour and about two to five centimetres in diameter and can be up to 45 centimetres long. That's long. Really long, and I'm going to suggest that a 45-centimetre stool would be some kind of world record. If you find yourself measuring one longer than that, I would call the record book guys, and you should also have a good think about why you have found yourself in a position where you are measuring poo. Anyway, it should gently slide into the water, not hitting it like a bomb, before gently sinking to the bottom of the bowl.

Unhealthy stools indicate a possible problem, the least alarming being dehydration, or a recent bad meal or a poor diet. The worst-case scenario would be an indication of a disease. You need to avoid finding yourself straining painfully or staring into lumpy pieces. If your poo is pale, white or grey, this could suggest a lack of bile brought on by hepatitis, cirrhosis or pancreatic disorders.

Just as the colour of your urine is an indicator of good or poor health, so the colour of your stool can tell you what's going on in your body. Another example might be yellow waste, which could indicate a gallbladder problem. And while this is no joking matter, there's the question of your poo's smell. If it's really, really bad (taking into account last night's tub of butter chicken followed by a bag of licorice bullets) it could be an indicator of certain diseases such as chronic pancreatitis.

So, while it might seem I'm speaking the obvious, I believe it's essential to drum all of this into your mind; knowledge is important and the more you watch and learn what's normal for you the better equipped you'll be to react when something changes.

PERSONAL HYGIENE

Your polite friends might grin and bear it, hoping that you'll step out of smelling distance. There's no getting around it—we all have body odour. Depending on numerous factors, it will just be a little 'whiffy' or quite overbearing. Time, then, to delve into this medical phenomenon which might influence just how tolerant your friends can be.

What I find fascinating is that we all have an individual odour—like our fingerprints—which is influenced by genetics. Perhaps in the high-tech future investigators will keep a database of odours which will help them catch crooks. A little gadget that captures the odour at the scene of a crime and this is then compared to a database. Linking the readings with fingerprints and DNA, the odour left lingering in the air will be evidence enough for a conviction. What the criminal has eaten might change the aroma, but the underlying, unique, odour will remain. To all the stinky felons—get ready.

But back to everyday life and the odour you produce. You can wash on a daily basis, convince yourself that your body is squeaky clean, but the odour is still there. You can't do anything to stop it. By stepping into the shower you've just managed to smother it for a while.

Impossible to stop it? Yes, but we can manage it.

First, it's important to understand that your body odour is undetectable by you in most cases, until it gets really whiffy. You might see a sweaty person sniffing at their own armpits and they'll just assume that because they can't smell anything bad there'll be no problem sitting in the audience at the opera or the cinema. You've probably been on a plane and gagged at the odour being emitted by the passenger next to you. Hopefully, they're not thinking the same about you! In any case, to avoid that happening, there are some rules that can help keep you on the sweet side of the odour game because you don't want to be known as 'that smelly guy'.

Some sweaty people's odour is more offensive than that of others. It's not the sweat that's producing the smell, it's the bacteria feeding on the sweat that are the culprit. There are more bacteria on your skin than you have cells in your body and they work at breaking down the proteins found in sweat. Those sweaty corners of our body—underarms, groin, feet—are breeding grounds for that active bacteria. It's in those areas, warm and moist when we sweat, that bacteria have a field day, putting you at risk of being socially undesirable.

When I say 'we' all have odour, young children don't have it, unless of course they haven't been toilet trained yet, but that's a different thing altogether. Body odour starts to develop later, as those kids grow into puberty, the hormones start to kick in. As adults, how we live and what we eat can change the composition of our sweat. For example, if we eat spicy foods the smell that comes from us is more pronounced. You can actually influence the way you smell by the food you eat.

One very interesting example I heard of was the airline worker who said he had become an expert at identifying where an aircraft that had just landed had come from by smelling the air around the exiting passengers. In many cases the air was thick with the aroma of exotic spices exuding from breath and skin.

If you're a guy with body odour issues, you need to do all you can to reduce food-linked smell. One way is to change your diet, cutting down on cruciferous vegetables such as cabbage, cauliflower and Brussels sprouts.

I appreciate that these are the same types of vegetables that are recommended as being cancer preventers. If you reduce your intake of these vegetables to reduce your body odour, are you then risking disease? It's all a question of balance, of moderation.

I should add that alcohol and caffeine will also make you sweat more and therefore smell more. But there are a number of other causes. Diabetes will make you sweat more (there is no simple way of explaining it) and there's also stress of both mind and body. Have you ever found yourself in a tight situation, the pressure is on and you get that sweaty, tingly feeling in your body? Up pops the sweat and its accompanying odour. I imagine a scene such as a businessman working late into the night, his jacket is off, tie askew. He's drinking cup after cup of coffee, gets up from the chair to pace up and down, all because he absolutely has to have a contract drawn up by the morning and it's full of problems. He's against the clock and all will be lost unless he produces. In that situation, I can almost smell that scene in the office.

Stress sweat in a circumstance like that tends to smell more than that produced from physical exercise or by temperature heat because different kinds of sweat glands come into play—there are different proteins that the bacteria will home in on.

Interestingly, dogs can tell when people are stressed thanks to their superior sense of smell. They can also tell when people have certain types of diseases. Research has found that there are some breeds that have a sense of smell which is an incredible 100,000 times stronger than that of humans. There have been cases in which dogs have been able to smell bad organic compounds in the body, their attention to certain areas of the body warning of a medical problem. A trained dog will pick up the illness through breath or sweat. I'm really hoping my dog isn't one of these specially trained ones, because if she is I definitely have testicular and anal cancer, and so does anyone else that comes to our house.

At the risk of stating the bleeding obvious, washing sweat-stained clothes, and not putting them on again before they've been cleaned, will help considerably to cut down your odour. Feet, socks and shoes are all wonderful breeding grounds for bacteria because it is there that up to 15 per cent of people have large amounts of sweat glands. Been for a run? Tossed your T-shirt, shorts and socks in the washing machine? All well and good but what about your trainers? Shoes are often ignored, yet every day that you fail to dry them out, by putting them out in the sun or leaving them in a well-ventilated place, the smellier they're going to get. And for goodness sake, don't wear any shoes without socks—this habit will send that bad bacteria straight into your footwear.

We have to sweat to let out body heat and through this natural process we are encouraging the breeding of little bacteria devils. We can't stop it, because if we didn't sweat we'd collapse as our body overheated. Sitting on the couch in a warm room watching TV will start to make you sweat. If it's not to an excessive amount you might not be emitting a heavy odour, but it will still be there. The same if you're too hot under the doona in bed.

People who have more body hair tend to be smellier. Sorry, it sounds mean but it's a fact. Hairy underarms create places for the smell bacteria and I can't overemphasise the importance of washing your hair on a daily basis. Shampooing the hair is generally underestimated by men. Dirt, oil and sweat build up on the scalp and in the hair and while this might not be an area where we sweat profusely, a good overall wash from the top of your head to the tip of your toes will all lead to a fresher you. Underarms, groin, feet—keep them clean while washing your hair.

The more obese you are, the smellier you are likely to be. Again, I'm not trying to sound like the mean guy. Facts again. All those folds of skin add to the problem. Those creases are perfect sources for odour and they're also easily missed when standing in the shower. So, by reducing your weight and you are also improving your chances of cutting down your odour.

Do you know what our biggest organ is? Our skin. On average, we have between 1.5 to 2 square metres of skin, making up 16 per cent of our body weight. Skin is something we take for granted. Its keeps all our other organs and blood neatly wrapped up, and protected. If it's not working at its best, the rest of us is impacted. I mention this to emphasise how important the skin is because it can influence everything from how we look, to how we feel to how we smell.

Not to generalise, but it's a pretty well understood belief women tend to be much better at looking after their skin than men. However, there is more of a shift in the younger generation towards making the care of skin and more meticulous grooming—manscaping—socially acceptable.

As long as you remember that it's not your sweat that smells. It's the bacteria feeding off the sweat that causes bad odour—keeping those microscopic devils at bay through cleanliness will help to keep your friends close and stop your partner grumbling about you.

BATHING

If you're anything like me you start every morning the same way. After your alarm goes off you lie in bed determined to unlock the secrets of the space time continuum so that you can spend an extra 10 minutes under the covers. I haven't figured it out yet, but I know I will. So, you drag your sad, sorry backside into the bathroom, and turn on the shower. As much as a hot, steamy shower is pure bliss, I advise you not to have the water too hot. You might think that the hotter the water, the more grime you're getting rid of but the reality is that a very hot shower will damage your skin. There's an outer layer known as the stratum corneum and it forms a vital protective barrier for the underlying skin. Too hot a shower and you run the risk of drying out that layer, washing away all the protective oils. Think about what happens when you lie in the bath or stay in the swimming pool for a long time, you'll notice that your skin wrinkles. This is a good example of the impact water can have on hydration levels in the stratum corneum.

And it's not just too-hot water than can cause this. Harsh soaps can also damage that outer layer. General advice gets tricky when it comes to skin, because different types of people with different types of skin need different types of cleaning products—makes sense I guess. It stands to reason too, that if you already have dry skin you need to avoid soaps with their alkaline consistency and go for watery washes, nothing fancy. A simple, regular routine of washing and cleaning yourself in as gentle, but as thorough, a way as possible, will set you up for the day. Well almost. There are two more tasks to fulfil.

You'll need to clean your teeth and whether you do it now, while you're in the bathroom with a towel around your waist or whether you do it after breakfast is a personal choice. Just be sure you do it. I'd recommend brushing your teeth after you've eaten, up and down, around and around, not forgetting the gums, and floss to search out all the gaps. Dental hygiene is not only important for oral wellbeing, it also impacts overall health. Recent research has shown increase risk of a cardiac event in those with poor oral hygiene. So, I don't want to treat you like one of my kids, believe me when I say it's become my most predictable battle of the day, but I have to ask 'Have you brushed your teeth today?'

MANSCAPING

Manscaping could very well be my favourite modern word combo ever. I mean, could you imagine being the guy standing there sculpting his beard into a topiary swan thinking there should be a word for this. If a man was a garden, his hair was foliage, and a razor a hedge trimmer, I would be landscaping a man, I would be manscaping—genius! Whoever you are, I applaud you.

For the wild men that enjoy a natural overgrowth of their garden, this section is not for you. For those that like to keep it in check its best to be prepared. Sharp blades near important things shouldn't be taken lightly. Anyone that has lopped too much off their favourite tree knows what I'm talking about.

Shaving is a very 'man thing' to go through, a scourge on the male population, and you do it because you have to. Gone are the days of the cut-throat razor—although some brave souls still use one—but you still have to take great care when shaving and not rush through the routine. The whole point of the exercise is to end up looking the best you can.

Your facial hair has an impact on your appearance. It can make you look or feel tired, give you a manly countenance, leave people wondering if you're a model or a criminal. Consider how a shaved-off moustache can leave people thinking, 'There's something different about Michael today but I can't place it.' You can also leave a stubble, manicured with an electric shaver. There's so much to face up to, if you'll pardon the pun, as you stand in front of the bathroom mirror.

Aside from any fancy appearances, let's deal with a simple shave, which in fact is not at all simple because there are different ways of approaching it. Your razor might have two, three or four blades, given the modern-day competition between razor manufacturers to see just how ridiculous you can be squeezing blades onto one razor, but it doesn't really matter how many, they just have to be sharp. You're better off buying a quality razor. Don't cut corners or you'll find yourself scraping and scraping away, harming your skin and still be left with a rough feeling as you run your hand around your face.

The best conditions for applying the blade are when the bristles are pliable through the application of warm water and thick cream or gel. Don't drag the blade against the grain, so to speak. Follow the natural direction of the growth and don't go over the same place twice without re-applying more gel or you risk harming the underlying skin, getting a rash or cutting yourself. There is also a danger of infection.

Shaving is not confined to the face. Chest hair and back hair are obvious targets for grooming, for some, arm hair, and leg hair as well. I'm not judging, I'm a groomer. Not an extreme groomer, and I'm genetically not a hairy guy. But I like to keep it in check.

Until recently grooming body hair was considered a very un-manly thing to do. And then along came metrosexual man and anything and everything goes. But as with shaving the face, applying a sharp blade to the body—and very sensitive parts of the body, too—has to be done with the greatest of care.

CAUTIONARY TALES

You will not believe how many men end up in the emergency departments of hospitals bleeding profusely because they've tried manscaping with their own hand. They've taken off a nipple, nicked a blood vessel on the scrotum and even the odd shaft slicing. Enough said.

What's this about the shaft and scrotum? Yes, if you haven't yet waded into the world of pubic maintenance, it is a thing. And why is that such a surprise. I think it's a bit rich to expect the fairer sex to use wax, laser and razors to keep everything in check but it's okay of men to present what could only be described as an unruly thicket of overgrowth.

A lot of men are opting for DIY body topiary, which isn't without its risks. Nick the wrong thing in that area and there is a very real in danger of either bleeding heavily or ending up with an infected penis. Badly-controlled manscaping can have a serious effect on sex life. It shouldn't happen to you because you have now been warned, but if the worst happens and blood flows and you can't stop it, apply pressure, grab a towel and get yourself to a hospital.

Trying to make yourself look good can go terribly wrong. You can end up looking the worse for wear. One young man I treated was suffering from a severe case of folliculitis (an inflammation of the hair follicles) on his back. You're no doubt aware that these are tiny bulbs at the base of every hair and in this case the poor guy had asked his partner to remove his back hair by waxing. The result was that he had suffered an infection and ended up looking like he had measles. By removing the hair, he had opened up spaces in the skin on his back which created an entry point for bacteria with the resulting inflammatory response. It's a tricky position for some men to find themselves in, being aware that their hairy body leaves them looking like they're wearing a bear suit, but removing it isn't always that straightforward.

What started this manscaping trend? Perhaps it's the influence of the ladies. Fifty per cent of women these days have shaved themselves completely. Some suggesting there will be an entire generation of men who have never seen a woman with pubic hair. The times are a-changing.

THE REALITY CHECKUP

Q: What are the elements of a good bathroom routine?
AR: Have one. That's the first thing. It just makes it easy to stay on top of things. It's good for your physical wellbeing as well as also your mental wellbeing. Keeping things clean and tidy means there is one less thing you have to worry about. Life has too many things to worry about but being unclean doesn't need to be one of them.

Q: What is a good basic rule for bathing?
AR: If you stink, bathe. Sure, that doesn't sound very scientific, but it's a strong starting point. There can be issues if you are bathing too much, but there are lots of issues if you stink too. Once a day should be a baseline, but if you need two baths on one day don't overthink it. If you don't believe me put it to the test. Don't bathe, let the stink build up and get back to me if it's working for you.

Q: What should I do if I notice any changes to my toileting waste?
AR: Consistent and concerning changes should be discussed with a medical professional. Trust your gut...literally and figuratively. Keep an eye on things so when there is a change you don't waste time getting it reviewed. Don't forget to apply some commonsense as well. A diet of beetroot and rhubarb will change things temporarily

Q: How do I talk to my partner about personal hygiene issues?
AR: If they are your hygiene issues, be honest and brace yourself for some hard truths. If you are trying to broach the subject with a partner the same applies—be honest and brace yourself. Would

you prefer to know if you stank so you could do something about it? It hurts in the beginning but it's better than spending your whole life as the stinky guy.

Q: Is being 'over-focused' on manscaping unmanly?

AR: Being over-focused on anything can be unhealthy, but calling something 'unmanly' is ignorant, and to be frank, the sentiment pisses me off. What is manly? Do you have to watch footy, have back hair and a beard? Do you have to crush beer cans on your forehead and regularly grab your own crotch? Absurd stereotypes and the use of narrowminded labels are exactly that, absurd and narrowminded. If you want to 'manscape' and take care of your grooming, then do it. If you don't, then don't. The most 'manly' thing any man can do is be man enough not to judge anyone else.

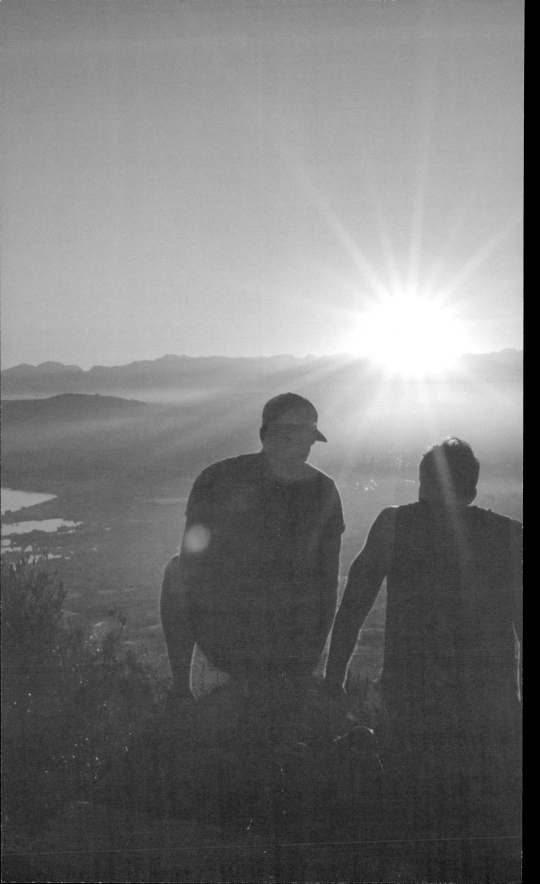

7. MATES

My best friend is the one who brings out the best in me.

Henry Ford

H ow males deal with their emotions in a mateship circle is quite important, and there can be significant impacts if you don't do it properly. It's really important to have close friends—we call our closest friends our mates. It's also pretty well documented that men aren't great at maintaining healthy relationships with other men compared to the way women interact with each other.

There tends to be a bit of superficiality as well as a level of unhinged bravado associated with the term mateship. The cliché is that we like to get together and drink and boast about our little triumphs, we talk about football and cricket...all that stuff is very important, but a lot of the time not much happens from an emotional point of view.

Social health, and I'm not talking about how many

followers you have on Instagram or Twitter, isn't something that tends to get a lot of press, but it is becoming more and more obvious that the lack of a healthy social life will start affecting your health. This is more apparent as we age and start losing our circle of friends. There's nothing like the death of a friend of your own age to make you consider your own health.

One of the positive aspects of alcohol consumption is when people drink in a way that is socially beneficial to them. They drink with friends, have good conversations, enjoy themselves and laugh together.

I think that we can start by looking into the impact of mateship on our health.

Firstly, there is no perfect number of mates that you should have. Having more mates than your friend doesn't mean that you have a healthier, more mature social life. It actually comes down to quality. We've found that the quality of your friendships is more important than the quantity of your friendships. There are some people who pick up friends along the way through life and keep all of them and they're very good at it. There are others who only have a small, close circle of friends.

As you age and as people change and go through different stages of life, it's actually very hard to keep close friendships. And the meaning of a close friendship for guys hinges on whether that friend in particular is a confidante, somebody you can turn to when you're not doing so well. Someone with whom you can share your most private thoughts.

Mates are really easy to have when the world looks

rosy. Mates are the guys that you're going to the footy with. They're the guys that you're hanging out with and having fun with. When you're at school and you have very little to worry about in life, you have lots of mates—you're all just kicking around. You're having fun, the world looks pretty bright, you've got food on the table and somewhere to live. You get into trouble here and there but you're having fun.

As you get older your life circumstances change. Some of you get married, some have kids, some lose their jobs, some have great jobs. Some of your schoolmates are making more money than others and it does start to put strains on those friendships. That's the difference between a casual friendship and a truly lifelong friendship.

You have to understand that, like any relationship, friends require effort. You have to work at maintaining social relationships. I can honestly say it's not my strong suit. Do I like being a good friend? Definitely. Am I good at being a good friend? I'm not sure that I am. It's important to be your own harshest critic, but it's also very important to understand that it's up to you to put in the effort. That means you have to figure out what it is that you're getting out of this relationship and what are you willing to put into it in return.

I think it's more about quality than quantity. I'm not somebody who needs to be friends with everybody but I am somebody who values really strong friendships—people who I don't necessarily speak to for a long time but I know are going to be there when I need them. In the same way that I will always be there for them. They, to me, are the really valuable friendships. They are my mates. And I think that all men need to have those types of relationships in their life.

The benefits of seeking good friendships and good relationships, whether they're centred around golf, basketball, touch footy, soccer, or work friendships, far outweigh the idea that you can't be bothered and you don't want to put up with other people.

Having a healthy social group of friends is really important, not only because we know it will help you live longer, but because you will also enjoy a better quality of life. And that's not only the good times—when it gets hard, you have a support group. People without supportive friends are often at risk when it comes to mental health and suicide. No life is perfect, and dealing with the inevitable ups and downs of life is much easier if you can share your burden with a friend.

I start by asking myself what that person means to me and then ponder what it is that I can do in return. If you're constantly taking from that relationship and you're not actually giving back, it doesn't work. You have to be open to the idea that you've got to communicate, you've got to give, you've got to be there when they need you, just as much as you expect their help when you need them.

It's about having a level of emotional maturity, and for guys that's not always easy to manage. You might be closer to someone in your group of mates than you are to the others. Egos can be easily bruised. You have to learn to manage different relationships all at once.

At the end of the day the important people for you are the ones with whom you can do the simple stuff, like having a beer and talking about absolutely nothing, right the way through to sharing the really difficult stuff with each other.

THE DARK SIDE

I'm pretty black and white on destructive friendships. You're not a friend if our relationship is destructive. I don't want to be friends with you if you are somebody that doesn't have my best interests at heart.

There is no perfect friend. There are times when your friend may not call you for months. You're sitting around thinking, 'What have I done wrong?

There is no perfect friendship but there must be, at the least, a mutual level of respect, understanding and trust in the fact that you've got each other's best interests at heart. They're not going to do something that jeopardises you. If they do, is it still a friendship? Are you still mates? Does this person care more about themselves or other people than they do about you?

I think that you have to make sure that the impact that they're having on your life is positive. These are people that you invite into your world, in the same way they invite you into their world. For them, you might turn out to be that destructive friend. You need enough insight to decide what it is about this friendship, this relationship, that is important. Ask yourself, 'What am I bringing to the table? Am I at any point taking advantage of this other person?'

Relationships of any kind—a sexual relationship, a

friendship, a marriage, a family relationship—can have huge negative impacts. If the relationship is adding stress to your life, if it's increasing the amount of anxiety that you're feeling, you need to really examine why you two are friends. Is it just because you've always been friends?

That emotional maturity that I've spoken about is just as important when you come to understand that your friendship or relationship is on the rocks—it's not working. A lot of guys struggle with being confident enough to just let a friend drift away. It's actually okay for you to drift away from a friend. You don't have to be friends with everybody that you were mates with when you were at school or university or an old workplace. And you certainly don't have to be friends with everybody that your friends are friends with. If there is something that makes you feel you don't want to continue in a relationship with somebody, that's okay.

Think about when you were exploring what it means to be a young man in your late teens, early twenties. I remember being put in situations by mates that made me very uncomfortable. It made me wonder, if these guys really are my mates, why am I being pushed into doing something that makes me uncomfortable? It's important to decide whether someone actually cares about you or whether they have another agenda altogether and you're just along for the ride.

It's okay to think, you know what, we're just different. We're not like we used to be. I don't want to do this anymore, and unless you want to just hang out, talk about stuff that I'm doing, talk about stuff that you're doing, actually enjoy ourselves out together and get something out of it, we're done.

Some people love staying out 'til five o'clock in the morning. If you're running in a group like that, that's fine. It just doesn't work for me.

Here's an important thought. I have friends who still like doing that, but they're my friends because they don't tell me that I have to do it with them to be their mate. They know who I am, I know who they are. We respect each other, and that's the important thing about any friendship, any quality friendship. There has to be a level of respect. We're not all the same. Everybody's different. People want to do different things at different stages of their lives. It's absolutely okay to say to someone, this is just not working.

It's important to understand that you have a set of values that evolves over time. Everybody has a set of values, that makes them who they are. You and your real friends will have a similar set of values. They will be the guys that understand. Yes, I'll borrow that money, but I'm giving it back to you tomorrow. And if you borrowed the money you will return it. If you screw up—no-one's perfect—you say sorry. If your friend is in the wrong, same deal.

That's how you decide who your real mates are and who are the guys who are just hanging on. The guys who are just hanging on are the guys that will have very different ways of doing things. That's the beauty of life. There are lots of different people out there. You shouldn't waste your time with people who treat you differently to the way that you treat them. Life is stressful enough without wasting your time on people that are aren't putting as much into your friendship as you're putting into them.

CLOSE AND CLOSER

As men, we are very good at having friends with whom we have a very superficial type of connection. These folks are very important people because a lot of the time they are the ones that we have fun with. Some of them you meet through sport or maybe where you work. You don't really need to catch up off the field or outside of office hours but they're your friend on the footy team or in the office. You need friends, you need colleagues, you need people that you get on with. But if they're the only types of friends that you've got, it's going to be really hard.

We all need those really close friends. We need to be willing to stand up and say, you know what, I really love my mates. My real mates, I actually...love them. They give me what I need and I think I do the same for them. We're not the generation who shake hands with their mates. I hug my real mates, because that's the type of relationship I have with them.

They mean so much more to me than a guy that I work with or even a guy that I've known for a long time. I think that we need to be willing to talk about mateship, because mateship is more than just saying cheers and yelling at a screen that's got footy on it. True mates mean more to us than that. I can guarantee right now, in the 85-odd years that you get to be alive, you're going to need those real mates, the really close mates, at some point. You're going to need them in the same way that they're going to need you.

Navigating all the relationships in your life isn't a straightforward thing. I think that if you go to an extreme that's a bad thing. Push all your friends away because of your partner—not good. Constantly hanging out with your mates and not spending any time with your partner—again, not good. Find a happy place somewhere in the middle.

I think a lot of Australian guys do one or the other. They do the big mateship routine—we're going to the races and I'll see you in three weeks—or they cut off their male friends because they get engrossed in the world of their new partner or wife. I think either extreme is unhealthy.

Finding the balance is the key.

THE REALITY CHECKUP

Q: How important to my general wellbeing is mateship?

AR: Social health is hugely important. In later life, those that remain socially engaged are more likely to live longer. We need friends to challenge us; to support, love, and help us, and to make us more accountable. Putting effort into friendships is just as important as putting effort into getting enough sleep, exercise and eating the right foods.

Q: Is there a perfect number of mates...too many or not enough?

AR: No. I like to think of 'true mates' like a movie—it's about quality over quantity. How many three-hour Hollywood 'blockbusters' have you sat through thinking, 'God, when will it end?' Well, if at any stage of a friendship you think that then roll the credits and move on with your life.

Q: Can mates be of either sex?

AR: Absolutely. I think women are much better at having male friends than men are with women, but what chromosomes someone has isn't on the 'mateship' checklist.

Q: How do I learn to trust mates enough to be vulnerable emotionally?

AR: You'll know, and the first time you are vulnerable will be a leap of faith, especially if you are mates that don't get too 'deep' when you hang out. There is a good chance the first time there will be a bit of initial discomfort but if it doesn't flow naturally and there is ongoing awkwardness then I'd reassess the nature of the friendship. It might just be more superficial than you thought.

Q: What should I do with a mate who has a negative impact on my life?
AR: Move on. Okay, sorry, that might have been a bit quick, and I know I'm probably overly simple in my view of such things. Let's look at it another way. If I was having a negative impact on someone else what would I want to happen? I would want them to be honest with me; to give me a chance to pull my head in and improve our friendship, or for us to then go our separate ways. There! That's a more reasonable approach. Then move on.

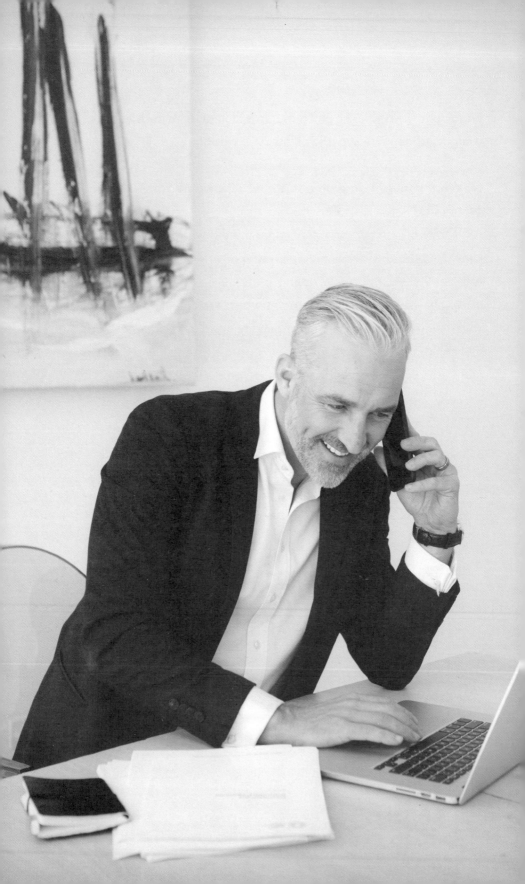

8. WORKPLACE

Choose a job you love, and you will never have
to work a day in your life.

Confucius
———

Work is something that everybody expects you should do. Just remember that on your eightieth birthday you're going to be looking back at your own life, you're not looking back at somebody else's life. It won't matter what other people think. And at that point, you really don't want to be thinking, 'God, I wish I'd done something different!'

Working lives and careers have evolved so much. It's no longer the case that you'll have one career. Nowadays you have the ability to have multiple careers over your lifetime and achieve so many different things. A lot of people say, 'I live to work.' Others say, 'I work so I can live.' Let's look at the whole concept of work–life balance and how we find it.

The starting point for me is purpose. Purpose is really

important. What is the purpose of what you're doing? What are the outcomes that you're trying to achieve?

When I was 20 I stacked shelves at a supermarket late at night. I was making money. It was a time of the day when I didn't have anything else on and I got paid to stick things on a shelf. I didn't have to think too hard. I pulled stuff out of a box and I stuck it on a shelf. It was a great job. My brother and I did it together, and the money I was making felt like a fortune.

The purpose of that job was to make money so that I could go out on weekends with my mates and have some fun. It was at a time in my life where it probably didn't matter but money was the only reason I was at work.

For most, work is a big chunk of your day. Actually, it's a big chunk of your life. I had other jobs when I was growing up too. As I previously mentioned I was an assistant nurse in a dementia ward when I was 17. I showered people, dressed them, I fed them. It was a hard job. I have the utmost respect for nurses or anybody who does that work. My mum pointed me in that direction. I always enjoyed that medical and healthcare space, so I took the job, but on one level I was still getting paid so I could go out and have fun with my mates on the weekend.

But there was something else. Every day was a challenge, every day was different. There were times when I did my job well and times when I did my job badly.

It was a fascinating place to be. And I'm not sure I fully understood that. I was doing things that I never expected I would ever do in my life; cleaning things up that you don't need to know about. It was fine. I didn't care. There was value in it for me as a person. Somebody else might hate that job, but I was getting more out of it than simply a pay cheque.

The dementia ward was like a time warp. Sadly, because they were suffering from dementia and Alzheimer's, the patients spoke to you as if it was the fifties or the forties, but I heard some fascinating tales that I really enjoyed.

There was Jock. Jock was from Glasgow, and Jock was a fighter. A trained boxer, who spent every day of the last years of his life reliving his days in the ring. He was in his late seventies, a five foot five ball of muscle. Too many blows to the head had likely sped his decline into dementia. When you walked into his room you had to be ready, because if it was a 'fight' day for Jock, you opening the door was like ringing the bell. He got me a couple of times. His jab was still solid. But my favourite memory was the day he wasn't happy with me standing there at six foot four. Jock started arguing with the nurse beside me that I was clearly not in his weight class. 'Who's this big bastard?' he yelled in his thick Scottish accent. 'I'll still knock his fucking head off.' Jock was a real character.

I started to realise that I wanted to do jobs that gave you more than a pay cheque. If I was going to give up part of my life every day, most days, then I had to get more out of it than money. There had to be a purpose.

And that can be many different things. For me, the value of going into medicine was being able to help others. I also enjoyed the challenge of highly stressful situations, never knowing what's coming through the Emergency room door.

It could be a multi-vehicle car accident or a boat accident or a young person with a brain tumour.

What you get out of your day-to-day job doesn't have to be what I value. You might simply enjoy working with the people around you. You may have work colleagues who like the same things that you enjoy. You all show up, have fun every day, laugh.

There's nothing worse than waking up in the morning feeling you really don't want to go to work. Many of us have been in jobs that are toxic. You don't have any worthwhile relationships with the people with whom you're working. You feel like an outsider, perhaps even physically ill. You don't feel like eating and you're stressed every day.

Situations like that are a great learning opportunity, a really nice insight into just how much your job environment affects your health. You have to be very careful about what work you undertake because it is part of your life. You leave your family, your friends, your loved ones on a daily basis to go to a job. If that job is making you physically or mentally unwell you have to have a really good hard think about what you're doing. Is the pay cheque the only thing you're getting out of this?

More and more science and research is showing that the level of satisfaction that you enjoy on a daily basis, especially from your job, affects how long you live. So, it's not okay to think, 'Fine, I got to the end of the fortnight. I've got my pay cheque. I'll do it again next week. I'll drag myself out of bed and I'll go and do it again.'

You can't ignore that stuff, not if you want a long and

healthy life. Sure, you need to earn a living, but it's important to understand that you need to work in an environment that is beneficial to you.

STRESS

Work is not without stress, but that can become a big problem if you're exposing yourself to an unhealthy level of stress on a daily basis. Acute stress is not necessarily unhealthy stress. In Emergency there was stress pretty much every second—category one, category two triage, let's get the room ready, what's happening here? Anything from a stabbing through to a car accident. That's acute stress. You need stress in those situations because it makes you think more clearly and make better decisions. That stress keeps us alive.

When you suffer chronic stress—you have a toxic work relationship, toxic boss that you don't like—when you're in a position where stress is a day to day to day thing, you start really affecting your health. Your stress hormones are elevated constantly, your blood pressure's up and your heart rate's up. You're revving your engine to the max for the entire day, to the point where you might not be sleeping at night because of anxiety about going to work the next day. You can get yourself into a feedback loop that is hugely detrimental to your health.

In health, being reactionary is the worst way to be. We've got a health system that is failing because it's set up to fix people when something's wrong, not prevent things from happening in the first place. Dealing with stress is the perfect example of putting in place a preventative strategy. If you are, on any level, starting to have physical symptoms as a reaction to a job, you need to ask yourself some questions. Does my job encroach on the rest of my life? Is it affecting my sleep? Is it affecting my other relationships? Am I getting home from work every day and pouring myself a huge glass of wine just to settle down?

If you find you've got no motivation to do anything else, you're exhausted, you're not exercising or eating crappy food every day just to try and make yourself feel better, it's time to take stock.

While it's (unfortunately) not uncommon for people under chronic stress to get to that point, it's only a problem if you let it continue to be a problem. You need to have sufficient confidence in yourself to be able to say, 'You know what? I'm not standing for this. This is making me feel bad and I have to do something about it.' That's step number one: recognising (perhaps even admitting) there is a problem.

Step number two is doing something about it. Sit down with your boss, sit down with your work colleagues, go to HR. Do whatever you need to do to resolve the situation. If you don't think that's going to work, it might mean you have to find another job. Is getting out of this workplace the only way to resolve all these issues?

Everything in life is a risk-benefit analysis. That's such a boring, scientific way to look at the world, but that's how it works. What are the risks of me quitting this job and finding another one? Maybe I won't be able to pay my mortgage. Maybe I won't find another job. Maybe I won't have the same friends that I've got.

What are the benefits? Well, if I'm not at this job anymore I won't have the stress associated with it. I'm potentially going to find something else that really does fulfil me. I'll be free to be able to decide what I actually want to do. And I won't be making myself unwell.

Some people work at simple jobs their whole lives and love it. They love the fact that they have no stress. They love doing their job to the best of their ability and they're nurtured by the relationships and by the sense of family and belonging they get at work. If the business closes down they're in tears. Everybody is different and meaningful employment means different things to different people. At the end of the day it's not about the job you do, it's about what you get from the job. Whatever you do it's important to enjoy your job and get satisfaction out of it every day.

Take some time to think about what you want to do. Talk to your friends about how their jobs go. You will probably have to change careers several times during your working life so try to be flexible. And there's nothing wrong with getting some extra qualifications—that will open up new perspectives.

Most importantly, will the job be purposeful?

Workplace dynamics are really interesting, like any human relationships. You're not going to get on with everyone. There are people who have a very different world view to you—they think differently. They may, for whatever reason, not like you. And you may not like them. That's reality. In most social scenarios, you don't spend much time in their company. You can get on with your life and never have to see them again. The problem with dealing with people like that in your workplace is that you have to show up every day.

You have to work out a way to manage that. The most obvious solution is avoidance, which isn't great, and in the workplace when you have to work closely with someone, is practically impossible. And you can't just ignore it. Don't ignore it.

How do you get to the point where the working relationship is something that is productive and not affecting you adversely? I think you have to be somebody who is big enough to understand that inflaming the situation isn't necessarily going to give you the outcome that you need. You also need enough insight to understand that if you're the person who is causing the problem, you need to change. It's a really tricky thing and every scenario is different, but you can't make everybody happy and you need to be true to yourself.

Sometimes you can't salvage these relationships. You have to develop a working relationship that is productive and achieves the things that need to be achieved. That means working with people who you just can't stand, who make you want to pull your hair out.

You can't solve problems by ignoring them. It goes back to something that I said previously in this book: your diagnosis doesn't change if you don't have the test. Avoiding getting the doctor to tell you what the problem is doesn't change the problem. If you have a problem with somebody at work, avoiding that fact won't make it go away.

In an ideal world, a one-on-one would solve a lot of issues. Another approach you might consider is having a meeting with a third person present. This is always good because the conversation cannot be misconstrued. But that doesn't always clear the air. And what if the person who is toxic is your boss?

You can find coping mechanisms, whether that is self-medicating with alcohol, becoming a recluse, crying yourself to sleep at night—whatever it is we all have our coping mechanisms. They actually get you nowhere. Well that's not true. They get you to the place where you are drunk, alone and in tears.

At the end of the day, what's the most important thing? I believe the most important thing is your health. Without your health, you cannot be anything to anyone else. Would you ignore a big, dark mole on your arm? Would you ignore chest pain and feeling short of breath?

The impact of chronic stress on your health is significant. Can you cope? Sure, a lot of us get really good at just pushing on. But the damage doesn't stop just because you have decided not to confront the problem.

You also have to decide how far are you willing to push the issue. But trust me when I say that a toxic relationship in your workplace can be the most toxic type of relationship that you'll ever have to deal with.

THE REALITY CHECKUP

Q: Can you put 'the workplace' into perspective for me?

AR: The workplace is exactly that, the place where you work. Work has a different role in everyone's life. For some, work *is* their life while, for others, work is about funding their life. For some, it's a good balance of both. Looking at work from a 'health' perspective, it doesn't matter what role work takes in your life as long as it's not impacting negatively on your health. Work can be both good and bad for your health—exciting challenges, gut-wrenching stress, great friendships and toxic relationships. Whatever work is for you, make it 'work' for you, not against you, when it comes to your health.

Q: What should I do if I feel I have no purpose at my workplace?

AR: Back yourself and change jobs. That may seem extreme, and I would encourage you to understand what it is you want to get out of your workplace and be open to talking before jumping ship. But I also think it's important to feel valuable; to feel you have a purpose and feel there is a reason to flog yourself at work every day. That's sense of 'purpose' is different for everyone but you shouldn't ignore the feeling if you feel you don't have one.

Q: How do I best deal with a toxic relationship at my workplace?

AR: A toxic relationship at work, or anywhere in your life for that matter, is bad for your health. Both physical and mental health. A lot of the time it can feel almost impossible to solve these types of problems but if it starts impacting on your health then you have to do something about it. Communicate, be honest, find support and do whatever it takes.

Q: What if work overtakes my private life?

AR: You have to define your priorities. It's up to you. There is no rule book on how much you should be focused on work and how much you should be focused on other stuff. It's up to you. Sure, your boss might think otherwise and to a point they are right—given I assume they are paying you—but when you start resenting the 'extra' you have to do and, in turn, stop putting in the effort then it's a somewhat false economy. There is a modern-day belief that you have to constantly do that little bit extra to get ahead, but the 'little bit extra' doesn't just rely on time, it relies on effort as well. If you're unhappy then your work will be unhappy and the outcome will make everyone unhappy.

Q: What is the best way to handle stress and anxiety about work?

AR: One: Recognise. Learn to notice when workplace stress is getting to you. When it starts to impact on your health go to...Two: React. If stress and anxiety has gone outside what's reasonable, you have to act. Three: Resolve. Ask for help. Take a break. Find the source of the stress and anxiety and set about fixing the situation. Stress reduces your ability to perform at your best. It impacts on decision making and harms all aspects of your health.

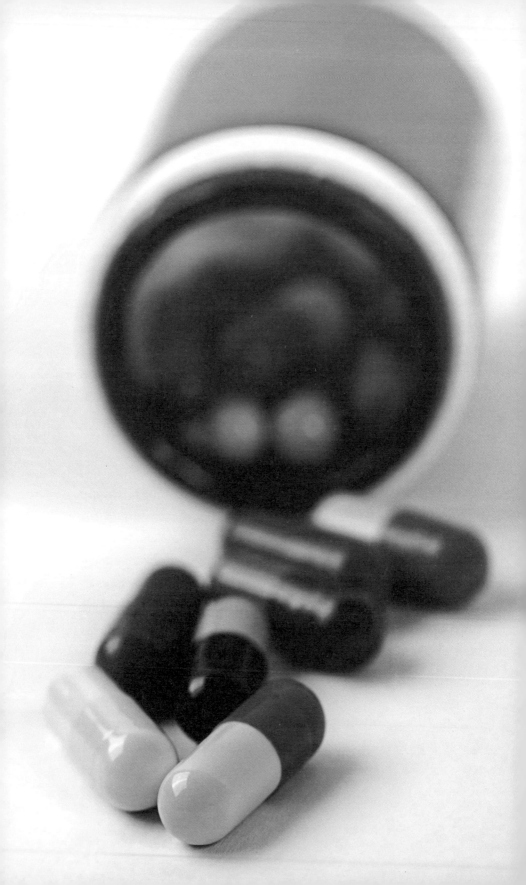

9. DRUGS

*All right, brain, I don't like you and you don't like me—so let's just
do this and I'll get back to killing you with beer.*

Homer Simpson

There are two major types of drugs. Those that will help
you medically and those that are used or abused for
recreational purposes.

In an emergency, you get to see the entire gamut of
recreational drug use. Most facilities have a special
treatment room. They're generally about three metres
square—not very big. One door, no window. All the
resuscitation devices you need are attached to the wall.

Patients who are combative or a danger to themselves,
you or others can be taken to this room so that you can
sedate them, restrain them and take the appropriate
measures to try and calm them down. Getting security
staff to come and help you calm patients down by putting

cannulas into their arms to deliver medication is a hard decision.

A lot of the time these are people who are acutely mentally unwell—aggressive, paranoid schizophrenics. People who have crossed the line. You're doing it for their safety as much as your own, and the safety of the staff around you, but it's never an easy decision to make.

Those rooms in an emergency department are most often used to deal with patients who have drug-induced psychosis. If they've taken methamphetamine (ice), a lot of the time they don't understand what they're doing. They get aggressive and they fight—really primal stuff—and the drugs give them an amazing amount of energy and strength.

One time we put a guy who was in the midst of a full-blown ice psychosis in one of these rooms to let him calm down. We left and locked the door (you can see through the glass) and walked away. When we came back he wasn't there. At this point you can understand the significant level of concern.

I swung open the door to see his legs disappearing through the ceiling. He had found a way to scale the wall, lift a panel of the ceiling and climb in. It must have been three metres up. The ability to do that, especially in that state, was just phenomenal; superhuman. He was trying to escape, convinced that we were some secret military group that wanted to cut his brain open and run tests on him. Paranoia is a very common element of all forms of psychosis.

WHY DO PEOPLE BECOME ADDICTED TO DRUGS?

There's a spectrum of addiction to drugs. People take drugs for a feel-good reaction—there's not a lot of point taking drugs if they don't make you feel good—whether it's the euphoria and high that you get from opioid drugs or the adrenaline rush and sensation of speeding up from amphetamines.

These are addictive-type sensations—you get addicted to the feeling that you get from the drugs. The simplest way to look at addiction is that it's the opposite to what you feel when the drugs aren't there. If you take a drug that makes you feel great and relaxed and calm and wonderful, when that drug is not there those receptors in your brain start crying out for it, making you feel anxious, tense and paranoid—you feel very uncomfortable. If you take more of the drug the feeling goes away. The more you use the drug, the more receptors you build, the more receptors you build, the worse the withdrawal symptoms are. It becomes a very vicious, addictive circle.

Some drugs are more addictive than others because they cause the euphoria and pleasant feelings more quickly. Addiction is a slippery slope because you get positive feelings when you take the drug, and negative feelings when you don't. The more you do the worse your addiction becomes.

HOW COMMON IS IT?

There is a pretty stereotypical view of what a drug addict is, but in reality, all kinds of people have forms of addiction. Anyone who's had a diet high in refined sugars and stopped eating them has a minor insight into what a withdrawal feels like. You're lethargic, you feel horrible, you get grumpy, you get angry.

Or try giving up nicotine. There are so many different versions of addiction. We've discovered or created substances, often for our pleasure, but you have to understand that if you use them, abuse them, there is a chance you will become addicted.

Basically, it comes down to management.

Often your circumstances dictate your relationship with drugs. The classic stereotypes being that unemployed people and petty criminals are addicted, but stereotypes are deceiving. Addiction is very widespread. And in many cases, we are unwilling to recognise that maybe 'I am addicted.' Some people have an addictive personality—they're more likely to become addicted to substances or they're driven by an obsession with feeling highs and lows. Lots of us don't know when we've had enough to drink or eat. Others are happy to go with the flow, happy with moderation.

It's not as simple as telling yourself, 'Oh no. It's fine. I'm not addicted to that at all.' There are chemical reactions occurring inside you that you actually don't control. Remember, no-one is perfect.

The notion that taking drugs is a victimless crime, that you're not hurting anyone but yourself, is not true. I think it becomes a really complex conversation depending on what drugs we are talking about. You have to remember that when people experiment with and use illegal drugs recreationally, they're breaking the law. It's risky behaviour.

In many instances people are trusting the unregulated manufacturers of the drug, and have no clear idea of the potency of the drug being taken. Relying on the people around them to look after them if anything goes wrong. And things can go very wrong.

I treated a uni student who had tried ice for the third time. This time his reaction to the drug wasn't the same as the last two times. He was found by paramedics in his room having taken his replica samurai sword and cut his own neck open. He ended up in Emergency and we had to stabilise him. It was a confronting situation, but we had to remain focused on one thing, getting him to surgery quickly so that he didn't bleed to death. He was very lucky that he missed all the major blood vessels in his neck and was still able to breathe. And that's a kid who was intelligent, had done well at school and got into university. By all accounts he'd talk to his parents and he wasn't a difficult child. He was just experimenting.

I tried a bit of pot when I was in high school. I was a real rebel. I remember being so concerned about what would happen I hardly even inhaled. It was so thoroughly underwhelming, it wasn't funny. It made me the opposite of the type of person that I want be—hungry and paranoid— and I didn't even feel that great. I had a lot of mates during that period who smoked all the time. I didn't see the point in that. I could understand the point of having a few drinks because you drank, you felt good, you had fun and everyone else was having fun. And I knew when to stop, so it rarely got to the point where I was drinking to excess. I sound like such a goodie goodie. Don't worry, I drank more than I should have on more than one occasion. I'll never drink Wild Turkey again!

I didn't get pot, and I'm not somebody who's experimented a lot with drugs. But I've seen people who never thought they would, break psychotically because of a drug. I've seen lives destroyed by addiction to recreational drugs, so I think I've been fortunate in a way to be exposed to the very nasty outcomes of drugs, and have a very real grasp of the risk-benefit equation.

Being addicted is a terrible lifestyle and no advertisement to try drugs at all. It feels good for sure—that's the point of drugs—but the reality is it changes your life forever.

WHY DO IT?

There is generally a reason people decide they want to take drugs. Sometimes it's simply experimentation, other times it's potentially mental health—depression, grief, or the desire to escape reality. Other factors come into play like peer pressure, and I think that if we want to solve this problem we've got to look more broadly at the issue. What is it that we aren't offering to the people that are doing this? Making drug taking a criminal offence is not working. It's not a deterrent.

Setting aside the people who profit from this industry and looking at the people that I would argue are the victims, I think we need to stop automatically making these people criminals and start understanding that there's more at play here.

Once people are on the slippery slope of addiction the fact that what they're doing is illegal is less of a problem than the impact it's having on them, their family and the people around them. A lot of the time people seek a simple solution to a drug problem that's not simple. It's a nuanced issue. For instance, many states in the United States have legalised the use of marijuana for medicinal purposes. I was involved with a very brave young guy who had bowel cancer. He was using cannabis to alleviate the effects of chemotherapy and treat the cancer. It was the only thing that worked for him. He was deemed to be a criminal.

As a society, we're beginning to understand that there can be a more sophisticated way of thinking when it comes to how we use, manage and police drugs.

As individuals, we ought to understand that taking drugs is not without risk—getting involved with any drug comes with a risk.

You can make a conscious choice to try something. That's fine. But you have to take responsibility for that choice. And understand the risks. There will be a flow-on effect to all other aspects of your life: your mental health life, your relationships, your ability to function in day-to-day life. Will you be focused, making great decisions, or will you be concentrating on what's happening this weekend, how you're going to get your hit? You need to understand that there are more aspects to using drugs than simply having fun.

I don't necessarily agree with decriminalising drug use; I think that's further down the track. If it was as simple as that—you have free choice and you are fully informed to make the decision—fine. But it's never as simple as that, whether it's selling cigarettes, drugs, or the types of food you eat.

I think you start by looking at the users and prevention. If you can stop something from ever starting it's a far better approach than letting a problem develop and then finding a solution.

PRESCRIPTION DRUGS

In the medical world, we try very hard to understand the interactions between medications and the patient, medications and the things that you eat, and the interactions between all the medications that you take. It's a precise if complex science.

Years and years of research, failures and successes, go into creating a prescription drug. It has to be tested in many different environments: tested on animals, then small groups of people, then larger groups. Does the drug actually achieve what we want it to achieve? What are the side effects? What does it interact with? What are the dangers?

Does the risk profile of this medication allow us to use it to treat a certain condition? These are sophisticated, complicated, very beneficial but also very dangerous substances. If they're misused, deliberately or accidentally misused, there can be serious consequences. One of the biggest reasons elderly people die is accidental overdose. And then there's intentional overdose.

Just because your doctor writes the script and you get it from the pharmacist and it comes in a nice package and is not sold to you by some dodgy looking guy on the corner doesn't mean that you don't have to understand the risks associated with taking it.

Accidents happen. People make mistakes. People think there's a pill to fix any problem without risk.

I'm trained in medicine yet I always make sure that I check the dosage of the painkiller that I'm giving to my child. I know how it works, I know the dosage, I know all that stuff, but I still check, still double-check. I understand the risks associated with most drugs. When used properly and safely and respectfully, the benefits are huge, but those caveats must be applied to anything from the pharmaceutical world.

Only take medications that are prescribed for you. Sometimes family and friends will say 'I've got some spare Penicillin or...' Mostly, the outcome's fine and that's a reinforcing behaviour. If you continue to do the same thing you're opening yourself up to something going seriously wrong. You become so relaxed that you apply those ideas about antibiotics to painkillers, then blood pressure medication, then diabetes medication...you can see where that might lead!

If medication is prescribed for you, the decision has been made taking into account all the factors that may affect you, not anyone else.

People can also become addicted to prescription medication. How does that happen? Surely your medical professional would know how long you've been on this course of antibiotics or painkillers. And yet, three years later you're still on the same painkillers.

Addiction to prescription medication is a very common thing. Opioids, Endone and oxycodones are simply a prescribed version of heroin. They make you feel good. Sure, they take away the pain in your knee, hip or your back. But they also make you feel good—euphoric and relaxed.

They are prescribed to address your pain issues. You have to understand that there is a risk of addiction associated with using powerful drugs like this. A very real risk.

One of the really interesting things about a lot of painkillers is that if you have a high level of pain you can absorb a large amount of pain medication. If you have a patient with significant pain you give them a huge amount of painkiller, it's fine.

But as soon as the pain goes away—the classic example is a dislocated shoulder or hip that is relocated—the second you have your shoulder or hip reduced (put back in), the painkiller dosage you've prescribed becomes an overdose. Because your pain has gone way down you can encounter all the other problems associated with taking a high dose of painkiller. You can stop breathing and lose consciousness.

You can see that if you're taking the same dose of painkillers for a long time, you've gone from solving a pain problem to making yourself feel good. If you continue to make yourself feel good, you get to the point where if you're not taking the painkiller you don't feel so good; you start to withdraw.

Sound familiar? Your brain creates more receptors for the drug, which makes you feel euphoric. When the drug is not in your system, the withdrawal's worse. You feel dysphoric, depressed, flat. You feel let down, so you go and find more of that drug to take away that feeling. And when that feeling gets taken away, you've found a solution to your problem and you continue to do it.

I've seen it all too often. Somebody who has a chronic condition has been prescribed medication, legitimately, for a very long time. They have a relationship with their GP or multiple GPs so there are no real red flags. But they're misusing the drug. They come to hospital and we have to treat them and we've got our own drugs that we want to use. We ask them what medications they're on and they just happen not to mention the fact that they are also taking high-dose opioids because they know they shouldn't be taking them. We give them medication without knowing what they've got on board, and...

I've been in situations where we've given people drugs that have put them into a coma, and then we're frantically trying to figure out why it's happening as well as reverse the effects. People need to understand that concealing this information is not safe.

People don't understand the interactions that occur. It all comes under the same umbrella: everything you put into your body affects you, that's why you do it. Alcohol affects your brain, the way that you breathe, your heart rate, your blood pressure, your gut. Medications have been created to affect various systems in your body. When you start layering them together, the risks go up.

Tragically, a lot of times it's accidental—it's a misunderstanding, it seems so innocent. By themselves, these substances are quite innocent. When you start taking a cocktail of different drugs you are running the risk of catastrophic outcomes. And you see it all too often, especially with the older generation. Some of them can't read the label on their medications correctly, or they take the wrong medication, or forget that they've taken their dose already and take extra doses and overdose.

Be careful. Don't be afraid to check. You can't be too careful with any of this stuff because if you misuse it, intentionally or accidentally, it can be very dangerous.

Last thought on drugs. I'd love to find somebody who has completely stopped drinking alcohol because they're taking some form of medication—it just doesn't happen. The best non-perfect way to act is to understand that there are risks associated with taking medication and trying to manage those risks. Create a monitoring process that makes you less likely to make mistakes, less likely to put yourself in a risky, harmful place.

It's the best way to figure out, the non-perfect version of you when it comes to drugs.

THE REALITY CHECKUP

Q: Is there any such thing as a safe level of illegal recreational drug taking?

AR: It depends on how you define a safe level? If 'safe level' means that you can take a drug without there being any risk of it negatively impacting your health, then that's naive. All drugs have risks, short-term and long-term. Obviously certain drugs have a safer 'dosing' profile than others, and at low levels may have minimal impact on your health, but there are others that have a very different risk profile. Those risks might be from the actual drug or from the risks associated with what might happen when you take the drug. Even prescribed drugs come with risk and, in most cases, there have been many years of research to find the ultimate 'safe' therapeutic level. But that still doesn't mean there are no risks.

Q: How do I know if I have a drug problem?

AR: If you are asking that question then that's a good place to start. Most of us have an understanding of when something is having a negative impact on our lives. Whether it's a job, a relationship or a drug problem it starts affecting relationships and people begin to recognise changes in you. You become fixated on getting and using the drug. Sometimes there is an uncomfortable physical and mental feeling if you don't have the drug and you ignore physical impacts, such as weight loss or weight gain, or even injuries that are occurring because of your drug use. At the extreme end of a drug problem you will find yourself doing things you never thought you would just to get the drug or because you are 'on' the drug.

Q: How do I challenge a friend who is abusing drugs about changing their behaviour?

AR: Be honest. Be a friend not a judge. And be there for them. Drug addiction and abuse on all levels is hard and sometimes people just need a friend to care and support them. But at the same time, you have to look after yourself. Not everyone is open to being helped.

Q: What is the relationship between prescription drugs and alcohol?

AR: By themselves, they both have risks. Taken together those risks multiply, it's as simple as that. Most of the time the outcome will be okay but that doesn't change the risk that something bad might happen next time. The other point is that if you are taking prescription meds then I hope that is for a specific reason. Alcohol, in a lot of cases, can alter the effectiveness of the drug and they don't work as well as they are meant to.

Q: What if the drugs I am abusing make me feel better?

AR: They probably do. That's the point. You have to decide firstly that you have a problem, and secondly, that you want to do something about it. Realise that the damage being done is far worse than the short-term feeling they might give you.

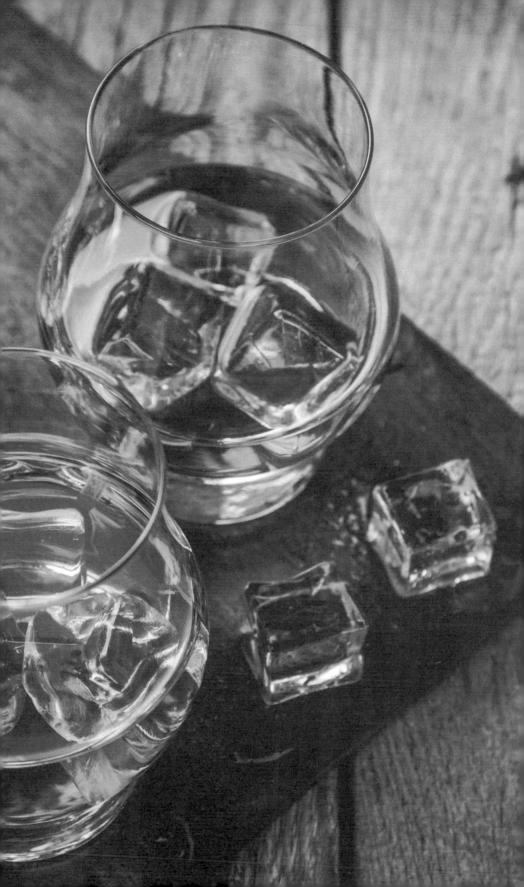

10. ALCOHOL

Pregnant women don't drink alcohol because of the effect on their developing child. No-one in their right mind would be comfortable with the risk of harm to the unborn baby.

The legal age for drinking is 18, but we can safely assume that younger people are imbibing alcohol. If alcohol is consumed by people around the age of 15 or 16 a developing brain is being exposed to a toxic substance. I'm talking about this as a scientist now.

It's also a really important stage of life, a period of time when you need to make some serious decisions. Do I get in a car with that friend? What am I doing with my life? What am I doing at school?

When I was a teenager I remember walking to a school dance after sculling a bottle of Wild Turkey in the park just outside the schoolgrounds. Me and my clever mate split the bottle. We were so cool. Acid washed jeans, a floppy mop of greasy hair and gangly legs and arms I hadn't fully grown into yet. I was one smooth dude. I think I may even have splashed on a bit of Dad's Old Spice—I wasn't even shaving yet! I just knew that I was going to have to beat the girls away with a stick that night. Little Dutch courage and I was going to be irresistible. Well it didn't exactly play itself out like that.

I remember walking past the teacher and I was fine. When I got to the stairs I couldn't walk up. The bits of the night I can remember were mainly of sitting in a corner of the room, staring at a wall to stop it from spinning. Needless to say, my dance card was the opposite of full that night. There was definitely no beating away with a stick. It was my first real experience with alcohol.

You do a lot of stupid shit when you're a kid, including making bad decisions about alcohol. It's really hard to tell someone of that age that his or her brain isn't fully developed.

When I was around 19 I was in a club, and there was a guy who was being very grabby to a friend of mine. She was really uncomfortable, and I could see her across the dance floor trying to catch my attention so I could help. Everyone was having a good time, and I didn't think it was too big of a deal for me to politely point out that she wasn't interested. He wasn't very interested in my thoughts, and proceeded to head butt me as I asked him to stop grabbing her. It took me a moment to realise what had happened. He was off his face. That's an understatement. He started throwing punches and I started to defend myself and we got thrown out. As I was complaining to the bouncer about not being let back in, I was king hit from behind and my face split open just above my right eye.

I was lucky, I was able to brace myself and prevent my head from hitting the footpath. He had as much time as he wanted to hit me as hard as he could. I still have a scar as a reminder.

Binge drinking is a serious problem. You are not just drinking to enjoy yourself, you are drinking to the point that you are so thoroughly intoxicated you put yourself and everyone around you at risk. Working in emergency I've seen more than my fair share of stupid shit people can do to themselves because of alcohol. Head injuries, a guy who scalped himself diving into the harbour, chopped off fingers, broken limbs, split lips, sexual assault, motor vehicle accidents, death—dealing with the results of intoxication is not fun.

One incident seems very fresh in my mind, probably because I still don't believe it.

It was a Saturday night like all Saturday nights. You get to a certain point and you just expect the accidents, mostly likely involving alcohol, to start rolling in. The usual practice in the hospital I was working in is that the ambulance guys who bring patients in after car accidents are asked to write up what happened on a whiteboard as part of the handover from ambulance to Emergency. What happened, how fast the vehicles were going, how many people were involved, what injuries were sustained. It was always an eye-opening experience. You learn the physics of trauma. Force equals mass times acceleration. The physics of an accident correlate with the injuries that occur. High-speed collisions between moving vehicles produce horrifying injuries to passengers.

On this Saturday night, we got the call that there had been a high-speed single vehicle accident. The young driver, intoxicated at the time, had lost control, clipped a parked car and launched into the front yard of a house. We received both the driver and young passenger. The passenger sustained significant pelvic injuries and was quickly stabilised and rushed to surgery to save his life. The driver had escaped with only a few minor scrapes. He had a blood alcohol reading three times the legal limit. As we were about to wheel him out of the resuscitation bay, he looked up at the whiteboard where all the details had been written and said, 'What's does the 150k mean?'

'That's how fast they estimate you were going when you lost control'

'Really? Wow, that's cool.'

Cool. He thought that was cool. You can imagine the look on my face.

That drunk little moron destroyed someone's car, nearly went through the front of a house and came very close to killing his mate. Yet he was still impressed that he had got the car up to 150 kilometres per hour. Young brains make bad decisions, add alcohol and the decisions only get worse.

HOW MUCH IS TOO MUCH?

I think you would be hard pressed to find someone who drinks alcohol regularly and hasn't misused it at some point. And that's mainly because it's a lot easier to misuse alcohol when it comes to your health than people think.

It's about how often as well as how much you drink. There are safe and harmful levels of drinking and the difference is not much. Alcohol is a drug and it does reduce stress but you need to give your body a rest.

On those days when you've had a tough time and you come home and drink, you are medicating yourself. The level of self-medication that occurs is quite scary. Some people say they have one glass of wine, but is it really one?

I'm not judging. I've done it, and I'm sure I will do it again. You stand there in the kitchen thinking about all the crap you had to deal with at work, the kids are squealing for dinner, your dog is barking, the neighbours' dog is barking, it feels like every dog on the planet is barking and you just want something to help you relax. So, you head to the cupboard reach past all the small glasses and grab the one with the capacity of a domestic swimming pool. You pour, you gulp, and you put down the meat tenderiser you were contemplating using on the neighbourhood's dogs.

In Emergency, when patients tell you how much they've drunk you mentally double it. You can have a few drinks most nights and go to work and everything is okay. What you're missing is the effects of chronic accumulation—persistent intake. You don't need to drink very much (if you do it all the time) before you start doing yourself harm.

Why are you drinking? Is it to escape something? Do you want to feel better? Are you anxious? Are you trying to impress someone? What is your relationship with alcohol?

You are not expected to be a saint, but it's best to avoid becoming a persistent drinker. It's very easy to become addicted to alcohol; you don't have to dig very far to find people who on paper would be defined as having a 'problem'.

THE REALITY CHECKUP

Q: What signs should I be aware of in the development of a 'drinking problem'?

AR: Again, like any negative behaviour, if you are asking that question then you may well have a problem. If it's affecting relationships, if you can't enjoy an occasion without alcohol and if you find you're constantly thinking about your next drink then you have a problem. If you are drinking at times you wouldn't normally drink, drinking to stop yourself from feeling hungover or drinking by yourself, these too are not good signs.

Q: What if alcohol is impacting on my home life or workplace?

AR: Alcohol had a way of creeping up on people. It helps reduce anxiety and stress, if only temporarily, but if you are 'self-medicating' then it can quickly become something you rely on to deal with more and more situations in your life. Other than the physical impacts on your health—increased risk of liver disease, bleeding disorders, cardiovascular disease, early dementia—it can also impact on your emotional health and your psychological health. So, be willing to ask for help; the difference between regular alcohol use, and functional alcoholism isn't as big as you may think.

Q: Can I enjoy a drink every night?

AR: You can do whatever you like, but is it good for you? You need to have 'alcohol free' days. The liver is an amazing organ; it can filter and metabolise so much of the crap we put into our body regenerate itself if its damaged—but only to a point. It needs to be given a chance to rest, especially from alcohol. So, alcohol free days are important. And it's also important to understand how your definition of a 'drink' fits in with standard drinks. I can confidently say, in most cases, we all enjoy an 'over-pour'. And why do you need alcohol every night? There is nothing wrong with a nice, social relaxing drink at the end of the day. There is a problem, however, if you swig it straight out of the bottle before you've even left the liquor store.

Q: How do I get my pregnant partner to stop drinking or smoking?

AR: It's really important that she stops, but that's often easier said than done. I definitely don't have all the answers but what I can say is you need to find help. The science is obviously no longer in question—alcohol and cigarette smoke are detrimental to an unborn baby—so, it's about helping her to stop for the health of the child *and* also for herself. This is one situation where the more help, including professional help, you can get the better.

Q: What if I am with someone who has clearly had too much to drink?

AR: Well, it's decision time isn't it. Do you leave them to wander around smelling of their own vomit, getting lippy with bouncers and generally acting like a drunken pratt? Or do you help them? I would argue that if you were a real mate you'd make sure they made it home safely because bad things happen when people are heavily intoxicated, really bad things. That said, if you are a true mate you'd make it pretty clear the next day that it's not okay to drink that much. We all make mistakes and lots of us push it a little too far now and then with the grog but drinking so much that you can't look after yourself is rather pathetic. When your main goal is to get as drunk as you can so that you need your mates to take off your pants and tuck you into bed, then you need to have a good hard look at yourself. I can guarantee you that those mates won't hang around very long if that's your 'thing'.

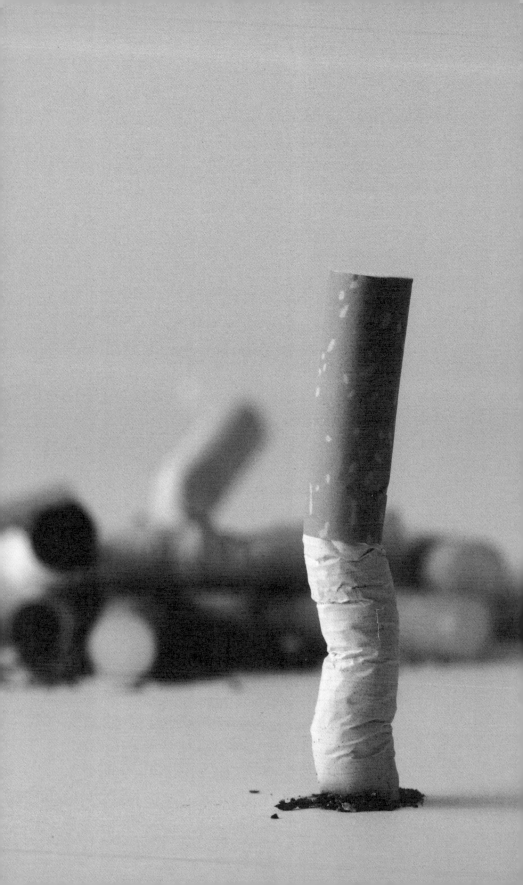

11. SMOKING

The message people should be getting about smoking has been very consistent now for some decades. The jury's in and the verdict is simple...don't smoke.

Smoking merely increases the list of things that we know will kill you. And unfortunately, there's no way to sugar coat that. There are things that we get told every day, we read about them in the newspapers and see it on the news, but when the latest research tells you that certain things increase the risk of cancer, or the chance of heart disease, or the risk of premature death, smoking is always top of the list.

Sometimes, the things that we think will kill us are based on weak evidence or early research or even 'fake' news. Remember the bacon scare recently? Talcum powder? Deodorant? Burnt toast? Researchers often find substances that are carcinogenic but such is the nature of medical science; it's all in the weight of the evidence.

And the weight of evidence is well and truly against smoking so if you are trying to find the best non-perfect version of yourself, when it comes to smoking the only thing

I can categorically say in this book is you need to be *perfect* at this. Don't smoke...even casually, socially or once a year... zero tolerance and zero intake. Nada. I realise if you are smoker we are probably no longer friends, but I can't alter facts. It is what it is. And you know I'm right.

We have long known now that exposure to cigarette smoke, even on a passive level, can generate cancerous cells in the body so why smoke at all?

If I can draw an analogy, asbestos is a good example. We now know that people exposed to asbestos have a real danger of developing a lung disease called asbestosis, the jury is no longer out on that one either. We know that exposure is directly linked to the development of mesothelioma and other cancers, so people avoid contact with asbestos at any cost. If you've ever renovated and had asbestos removed from your house you know what I'm talking about. It's like something out of an *Alien* movie. Spacesuits, watering, thick black wrapping plastics, disposal protocols; it's no joke.

Smoking is the same, without the spacesuits. Exposure at any level is harmful to your health. Whether you are a heavy smoker, casual smoker or passive smoker the dangers are real and so smoking is no longer socially acceptable. Although it's only been outlawed in clubs and pubs in Australia since 2006, it was just so foreign to me to be in Indonesia recently and to be asked in a restaurant if I would like smoking or non-smoking dining.

The developing world is still catching up to the ills of smoking in public places, but the scientific community has been on the same page for decades now. Smoking kills.

In saying that, however, I have a lot of sympathy for people who smoke because quitting the habit isn't easy. And for people who have a nicotine addiction it's obviously enjoyable for them to have a cigarette: they feel better when they smoke and they feel bad when they don't. As a doctor, and a human, I get that.

But the truth is, cigarettes have been created to deliver an addictive drug—nicotine—directly into our nervous systems. How cruel is it for a company to create something so bad for you that is also so addictive? And produce it legally as a saleable product and on a mass production scale? I'm sure some lawyers will have to make sure those statements don't get anyone I trouble. And I can't prove intent. But cigarettes piss me off. So, whatever.

There are many reasons why people smoke, but one of them is not ignorance. I just can't believe that there is anyone out there anymore who believes smoking is good for you on any level or doesn't cause cancer.

Obviously, there is peer pressure in certain age groups; you start smoking at a vulnerable age and when you get addicted it's a hard habit to kick. Maybe you don't want to stop smoking, and at some stage you may feel you are not at risk because you're going through your 'bulletproof' stage, but if you're asking my opinion as a doctor about smoking, just don't do it. And as a friend or a mate, the answer is still the same. Don't do it. As a fellow human being? Don't do it.

In fact, if you do smoke, do whatever it takes to quit. Seek medical help, ask your family and friends for support to try and get through it. Understand that it is going to be hard, understand that there will be times when you fail, but start now. Don't wait.

The good news, if that's the right term, is there is no perfect way to quit smoking. There are literally hundreds of different options you can take: commercial products, nicotine replacement therapy, hypnosis or just going 'cold turkey'. For each person, the 'perfect' way to give up smoking will be different.

But know that you'll probably fail at some point in the process. You'll have a tough day at work, someone will be smoking socially and you will 'fall off the wagon', just like any diet you may be on or fitness regime you might be trying to adhere to. There will be days when you fail but that doesn't mean you give up. Keep going. One step at a time and you'll get to the top of the stairs.

You have to be motivated to succeed: you just don't want to smoke anymore, you don't want to live that life anymore, or you want to take advantage of the many health benefits of not smoking; to live a life where you can breathe freely and exercise, and enjoy life fully with people you love. That should be motivation enough but whatever the reason, don't smoke.

This book is meant to be honest but also to be blunt; I have looked after too many people who have suffered from smoking induced lung disease in my medical career. We will all die at some stage, but emphysema is just a terrible way to die—literally spending the last years, months, days of your life gasping for air. And any one of those people I cared for—good, kind, loving people—would tell you the same thing. Don't smoke.

There are obvious long-term benefits to quitting smoking, benefits related to your skin, to ageing (cigarette smoking causes premature ageing), decreasing your chance of heart disease or dropping dead of a heart attack, reducing damage to the walls of the arteries and blood vessels that go to all the extremities of the body: your fingers and toes and your penis. If you care about those things—I know you care about your penis—if you don't, you have bigger problems, and the fact alone that damaging the small blood vessels that allow you to have an erection should make you want to give up smoking.

If you don't quit smoking, one thing is for sure, you will get to a stage in your life where you have damaged your lungs so badly that you have no quality of life left. If anyone ever asks me about health issues I tend to be very pragmatic, use a commonsense approach and bring some balance to the argument, but in truth there is no balance in the smoking debate.

Don't smoke. It's like falling off a cliff really slowly.

THE REALITY CHECKUP

Q: Is there a 'safe' level of smoking?

AR: No. Passive or active smoking, there is no safe level. The chemicals in cigarette smoking are toxic and cause cancer. End of story.

Q: Is giving up smoking hard?

AR: Yes...exceedingly hard. Nicotine is one of the most addictive drugs on the planet so understand that the pleasure you get from smoking is actually the feeling of not withdrawing from a drug dependency. That's a very vicious cycle to get yourself in and the only way to get out of that cycle is to go through a process of withdrawal.

Q: What if I fail?

AR: It doesn't matter. You probably will fail at some point but start your 'quit' contingency plan knowing that. Make it part of your 'quit strategy'. Even if you are motivated to quit and surround yourself with the right people and arm yourself with the right advice, there will be days that are harder than others and you may 'fall off the wagon'. But you only fail on that day, not in the long-term goal, so keep going. If it is the first time you have had a cigarette in a week, you are still seven days in front of where you would be if you had continued smoking.

Q: What are the immediate health benefits of quitting smoking?

AR: From the first day that you stop smoking you give your lungs the chance to start recovering and you stop the destructive process that has a cumulative effect on your health. Every day you smoke you increase the destruction of lung tissue, and you move further away from the ability of your body to heal itself. If you give up soon enough you can give yourself time for your lungs to return to the state of a non-smoker.

Q: Can I recover my full health if I give up smoking?
AR: Yes, but there is a time frame associated with that decision. You have to give up early enough to give your body time to recover but you also have to give up early enough so that your body is not suffering from the cumulative effect of smoking. The latest research says that if you give up smoking at age 30 you can have an identical life expectancy to non-smokers, so do it now. Smokers who quit between the ages of 45 and 54 gain about six years extra life expectancy. So, what are you waiting for?

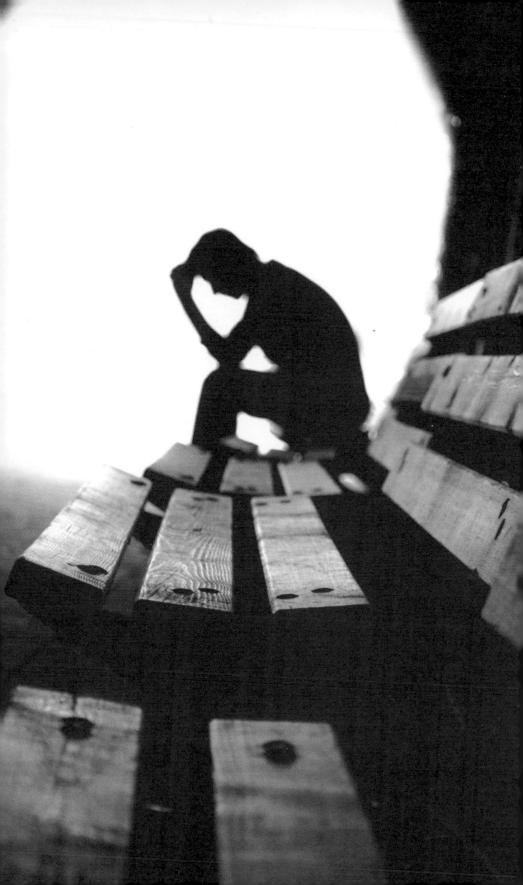

12. MENTAL HEALTH

Mental health has always been an important issue in your overall health but only recently has it received the priority it deserves. There's probably a couple of important reasons why we are hearing more about mental health issues now.

The first is that we are more open to hearing about mental health today. One of the mistakes we made for a very long time was in not recognising mental health as the same as other physical ailments. It's very easy for us, for example, to understand what a busted knee is, right? It's busted. You've hurt your knee, and now it doesn't work so well. Its functionality is no longer what it should be and there is pain there, you limp around a lot and the knee doesn't do what it's meant to do. It's a dodgy knee.

Mental health is the same. We have a series of connections in our brain that release a whole series of neurotransmitters in concert with each other that make us feel what we feel: make us sad, make us happy, make our personality and how we deal with certain situations. And everyone is different, that's why we all have such wonderfully different personalities.

For some people, areas of the brain are 'busted' and they don't work as well as they need to. People are not getting the neurotransmitters at the right time in order to function and so that part of who they are, that physiology, is not working at an optimal level.

Sadly, for a very long time, the response to mental health issues was 'It's all in your head!' or they were dealt with in asylums and not given the level of prominence needed. Thankfully, the stigma associated with mental health is slowly disappearing and the generally accepted understanding is that mental health is something that can be diagnosed, treated and managed the way an injured knee is diagnosed, treated and managed.

Another reason for seemingly increasing prevalence of mental health issues is that potentially we are creating social environments in which we are more at risk of developing different forms of mental illness or augmenting the ones we already have. Unfortunately, the nature of social media, increased use of technology and unrealistic expectations make us feel worse about ourselves than we should.

Workplace pressures, family pressures and financial stress all play a role. The expectation of extra working hours and what you need to do to 'get ahead' in the world, are not new problems. They have been around for decades and decades but I think in the past if they manifested themselves as some form of mental illness it wasn't necessarily treated or dealt with the way it is today.

So, we're seeing mental health issues more and more today but it's not a new phenomenon. I think we're more open about it and willing to talk about it but we still have a way to go for full acceptance, especially with men.

Men have never been great at tapping into our emotions (although that can be a gross generalisation) but it's a very simple and pertinent way of saying that we need to be open to having an honest conversation with those who are closest to us—our mates, our partners, our families—that you may not be yourself, that you're struggling.

And it's not just another tough day at work or that you're feeling flat. It's admitting that you are not yourself and you're not getting the full enjoyment out of life that you should be. You don't have the desire or motivation at work anymore; you're sleeping more, drinking more, withdrawing from the world or partying way too hard and are no longer doing the things you used to enjoy.

These are all red flags. You're not just having a tough day. You're not just in a rut. Your heart is racing, you have sweaty palms, and you can't sleep at night; we all have to be sure that we are not ignoring the signals. When they start happening consistently to you, you need to talk to someone about it. The beginning point for good mental health is recognition of a problem.

Stress is a form of mental health. Everyone has a telltale sign that something is wrong and they might be struggling mentally and emotionally. They might be someone who eats more, or eats less, sleeps more or sleeps less, drinks more, they might have a racing heartbeat and chronic headaches, and are just not interested in anything anymore. These are physiological signs that your mind, and therefore your body, is not working right.

Understand that there is nothing you can actually do about it until you talk to someone and seek a professional diagnosis. Mental health is not something you can talk yourself out of. Having seen some of the most heartbreakingly extreme versions of mental health—schizophrenic, psychotic breaks from reality—this is just not possible. Sorry. It's not.

I once looked after a man who presented to the emergency ward as an exceedingly successful businessman—immaculately well-dressed, with a coat and tie, carrying an expensive briefcase. The police had brought him to hospital after finding him wandering around the city. He was suffering from severe paranoia and believed everyone was involved in a conspiracy against him, listening to him on secret devices. He didn't trust any of the medical staff and thought the police were taking him to a concentration camp. It was very sad.

Now, to the outside world it was all exceedingly irrational, but take a moment to use your rational brain to understand that an irrational brain can't think rationally. It's a bit of a mind bender, but that's kinda the point. His brain no longer had the rationality to comprehend how irrationally he was acting. The truly mentally unwell don't understand they are unwell.

Many people who are mentally unwell have a genetic predisposition to being unwell but a lot of the time it is precipitating factors such as a traumatic life-related event such as grief, loss or ill-health that triggers a mental health episode. Chronic drug abuse is another.

We are each a very fine of balance of physical and mental issues that we'll never fully understand, and some of us are closer to the edge of tipping over than we realise. No matter what that balance is, we all need to understand that if we are going through it ourselves or helping a loved one through some bad times, just as you don't tell someone with a busted knee to run faster, it's pointless to tell a person suffering from mental illness to 'be happy'. They simply can't do it so at that point you need to be doing everything you can to get help.

Telling someone to just get better doesn't help anyone. They need proper medical help—diagnosis, treatment and a management plan.

The cruel reality of mental illness is if you try and fix it yourself, you're trying to fix it with something that is not working. If you've busted your hand you don't try and fix it with the same broken hand. And yet we sometimes expect people who suffer from a mental illness to do exactly that—fix themselves with the same broken thinking.

There are plenty of flat days, hard weeks and the odd mid-life crisis to navigate, and everyone experiences those things to a certain degree. Where am I going? What have I achieved? What does my life mean? We all experience those sorts of crises in our lives and there are differing opinions whether these are milder versions of mental illness or whether you are just in a momentary state of sadness. And there is a difference between sadness and depression.

While it may not be as easy as having a blood test for a virus, there are ways for doctors to figure out what is wrong, but you must seek professional help. The good news is in the past 30 years the medical profession has gotten much better at diagnosing mental health issues.

There is a lot misuse of mental health terms today— depression, anxiety, melancholy—in the social media space we've created and they can be terms that we just throw around, 'Oh, I'm so depressed,' and similar. We need to understand that clinical depression is a diagnosis by trained experts, not a catch phrase or a label to place on ourselves or others. We have to be careful how we describe ourselves and others, as do the media. The media is actually a key factor because that's how we can learn and understand about these issues.

The reality is you will not experience life without encountering a mental health issue at some point, whether it's you, someone you know or someone you love. The good news, if that's the right term to describe mental health, is that social stigma is lessening. It is now socially acceptable to say, 'I am not doing okay,' which is encouraging. The only way we are going to improve as a society is to make it easier for people to put their hands up and say they need help.

A lot of people are still scared about mental illness and identifying with one...what will happen to me, or to my relationship or my job? But also know that it is no longer okay for mental health issues to impact on your physical health, your relationships or your career.

Communication is an important starting point is seeking

treatment. Being open enough to talk to someone about it is important, as it is being able to listen to someone who has a problem. One of the most valuable things you can give someone is your undivided attention, especially at a time when someone is struggling mentally. There is no better gift than your time.

Suicide is a scourge of modern society. It's quite a dark thing to talk about suicide, but the message I try and get across is that suicide is *real*. I lost two medical colleagues to suicide. Sadly, we have a high rate of suicide in the medical profession—and these are people who are fully equipped to understand mental health issues and the impact of death and suicide on other people.

The one thing I tell everybody is if you think there is a niggling little voice in the back of your head, or a knot in your stomach, or something makes you feel afraid that somebody you know may harm themselves, then do not ignore it.

If you ask someone if they are okay, or the tougher question about if they are considering harming themselves, they may be upset with you briefly, but they'll brush it aside and later understand that you care enough to ask.

The other scenario is to say nothing and the worst might happen.

It may be a subliminal sign but you've seen it for a reason; they might have shut down for a reason; they might not even seem depressed. But mental health is a really tricky subject. They may be a partner, a family member, a friend or a work colleague, but if the idea even crosses your mind that they might harm themselves please act.

Given those options, you just have to ask the question.

If you have suicidal thoughts you have to get help. At some point in our lives we may have those dark thoughts, but the simple truth is you should talk to someone and see someone. I've had those days too, and uttered that throwaway line it might be easier to fall asleep and not wake up tomorrow, but it's not normal. Life shouldn't be like that and you shouldn't think like that. Please. Believe me when I say that there are people that care. If I can admit it here in this book, then I hope you can admit when you need help. Don't feel alone.

I am not as wise as I might be with a little more experience under my belt but the one thing I've learned in my 37 years is life is pretty simple, you have to enjoy life. You need to bring joy to others and to yourself so if life is treating you poorly and you're thinking you can't deal with it anymore you need to know that you may be thinking that for reasons you don't, and can't, fully understand, so seek professional help.

There may not be a simple solution to your issues but don't be afraid to ask for help. Everything is easier with help.

Who do you speak to? Start with the person you are most comfortable being vulnerable with. Reaching out when you are genuinely at your lowest is very hard, especially for men. That's why you need to have quality relationships around you (see Chapters 8) so you can feel comfortable with speaking to a friend of a partner or family members.

How do you get people to understand they have a mental

illness? That's the cruelness of mental illness. You have to give yourself the best chance to get better and that's by allowing someone else to help you.

THE REALITY CHECKUP

Q: Who should I talk to if I'm not feeling well?

AR: Top of the list is a trained professional and that's why you need to develop a secure relationship with a GP you can trust. Our health system today doesn't necessarily support the idea of the family doctor who treats generations of the same family. In years gone past, the family doctor was someone you could relate to, unlike the medical centres of today where you are trying to unload your thoughts to a complete stranger. So, find a doctor who you feel comfortable talking to.

More than that, have one or two people in your life you can be vulnerable with. It doesn't have to be a Rolodex list of people, but it may be a partner, a friend or work colleague. It may not be the obvious choice but it should the person you could ring right now and say, 'I'm struggling, I think I need some help...' without flinching.

Q: What support networks are open to you to receive the help you need?

AR: Lifeline 13 11 14

Black Dog Institute (02) 9382 4530

Beyond Blue Support Service 1300 22 4636

You need a referral from a GP, but there are free counselling sessions available on a standard Medicare rebate for most Australians.

Q: What if I am labelled or stigmatised if others find out I have a mental illness?

AR: Given that it may or may not happen, you cannot use that as a reason *not* to seek professional help. If it does happen, it says more about the people around you than it does about you. I think you will be refreshingly surprised how supportive people will be of your situation, so don't box at shadows that might not be there. You'll get the support you deserve. You have to ask first.

Q: Can people with a diagnosed mental illness still function effectively?

AR: 100 per cent yes. Most likely you interact with a number of people who do just that every day of the week. They either have previously, are currently, or will in the future, seek medical assistance for a mental health issue and are functioning effectively in their jobs, at home and in wider society.

It's like every other medical issue, it can be diagnosed, it can be treated by a health professional and it can be managed. Are there people out there who have had heart surgery? Can you identify them by working with them or talking to them? They had an illness and sought effective treatment and that's how we need to perceive mental illness.

Q: Will my diagnosed mental illness improve or will it be with me forever?

AR: People with a mental illness which is easily managed, or even those with a chronic mental illness, can lead a normal life with a supportive health management plan. There are so many variables but people rarely 'grow out of' a mental health condition, they effectively manage the problem.

It depends on the severity of the mental illness and the professional diagnosis. It's a tough one to answer, but your health professional will discuss with you whether it's a short-term ailment or

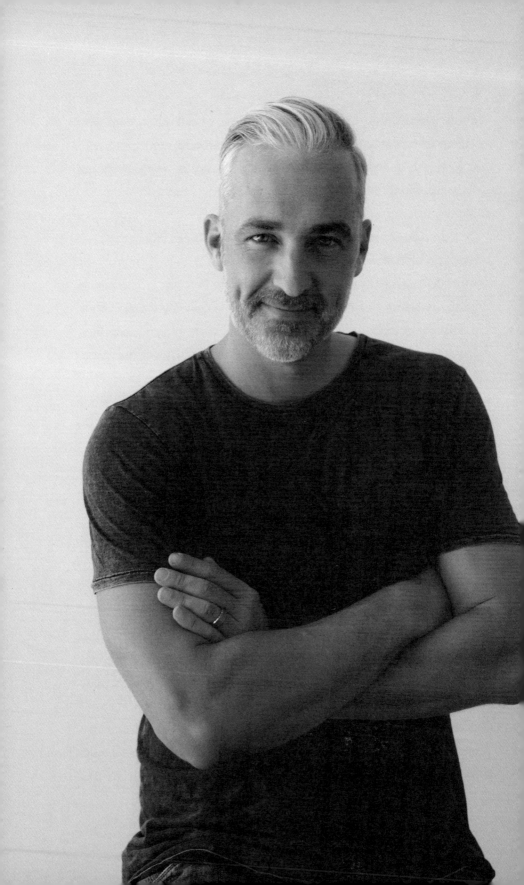

IN CONCLUSION

Having read this book I hope that you realise that there is no road map to perfection in personal health, and that I don't have all the answers.

I hope now that you've reached the end of the book you've been encouraged by the things you have read, and affirmed in the good things you are already doing. Recognise the things you might be interested in doing in the future and learn about the positive changes that you can adapt into your everyday life.

Combined, they may just tip the health scales in your favour so that you become a little healthier than you were at the beginning.

My goal for anyone who reads this book is to be slightly healthier by taking on some of these tips than you were at the beginning. Who knows what that may be? Perhaps its having a better understanding about your own health than you once had, of how you want to eat and how you should exercise and how you feel generally about yourself.

Above everything else, the one message I want to impart

is be comfortable in the fact that we are all individuals and there is no one book, or diet plan, or exercise product that will solve all your health issues. There is no 'one-solution-fits-all' approach to perfect health, because 'perfection' does not exist.

So, by taking the approach that perfection does not exist, the goal then is to become the best non-perfect version of yourself so you won't set yourself up for disappointment, and ultimately you will achieve more.

My hope is that you will make decisions and actively live a life that's more healthy without really knowing it. That's the real trick—not to get up in the morning with an impossible plan in your head of all the things you need to do to be healthier, but to get up in the morning and enjoy life and live it in a healthier way.

By embracing the best non-perfect version of yourself, you'll enjoy life more and hopefully have more of it. After reading this book you can't argue that there aren't many benefits to being healthier. And you won't have all the associated angst that comes with trying to achieve perfection.

There is no such thing.

To Archie James, Georgia Claire and Ava Rose,
for your hugs, your giggles, your kisses and your love.
Perfect in every way.

ACKNOWLEDGEMENTS

Special thanks to my wife Jamie, parents Michael and Trish, and all my family for your encouragement, support and patience in the face of my endless rants, crazy ideas and constant overthinking. Also, to the team at New Holland Publishers for all your hard work in making this book happen.

Lastly, to all those that have, and continue to, inspire me, it's a gift I hope to one day repay.

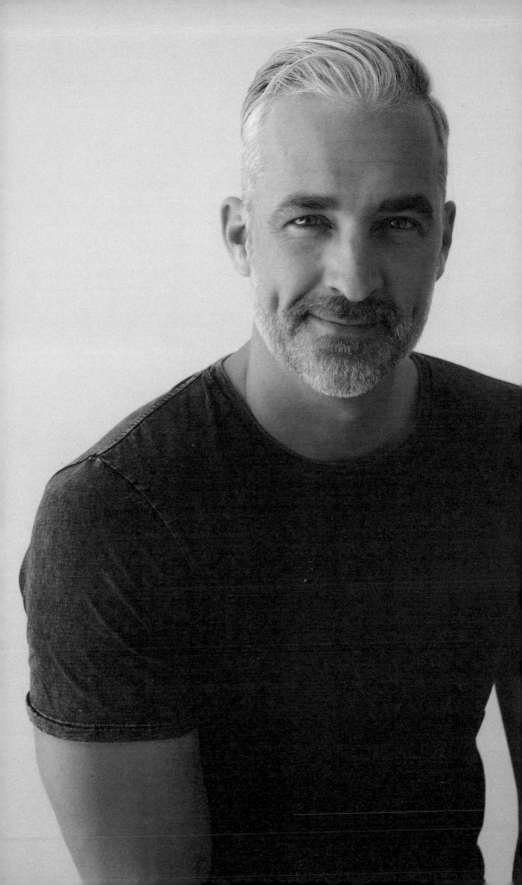

ABOUT THE AUTHOR

Dr Andrew Rochford is one of Australia's most popular media personalities and medical health experts, best known for his appearances on Channel's Nine's *The Block* and *What's Good For You*, as national health editor for Channel Seven and on *The Project* on Channel 10. He is an authoritative voice on current health practices, especially health issues facing men.

First published in 2017 by New Holland Publishers
London • Sydney • Auckland

www.newhollandpublishers.co.nz

The Chandlery 50 Westminster Bridge Road London SE1 7QY United Kingdom
1/66 Gibbes Street Chatswood NSW 2067 Australia
5/39 Woodside Ave Northcote Auckland 0627 New Zealand

A record of this book is held at the British Library and the National Library of Australia.

ISBN 9781742579658

Group Managing Director: Fiona Schultz
Publisher: Alan Whiticker
Editor: Liz Hardy
Designer: Catherine Meachen
Production Director: James Mills-Hicks
Printer: Hang Tai Printing Company Limited

10 9 8 7 6 5 4 3 2 1

Keep up with New Holland Publishers on Facebook

www.facebook.com/NewHollandPublishers

UK £14.99
US $24.99